ALL THINGS POSTPARTUM

RECOVER EMOTIONALLY AND PHYSICALLY,
REDUCE THE STRESS & ANXIETY OF
MOTHERHOOD, BUILD A SUPPORT SYSTEM, AND
NURTURE YOUR BOND WITH YOUR BABY

JOHAIRA MICHELLE DILAURO RN, BSN, CLE

ILLUSTRATED BY
IZABELLA XIOMARA DE LEON

To every mother stepping into the sacred, messy, and life-altering journey after birth — this book is for you.

*To my son, Nikola — you are my wildest dreams manifested.
Thank you for expanding my heart in every direction, teaching me patience, and deepening my ability to truly absorb the present moment.
You are Sparkle in Living Form.*

*And to my husband, Eric Dilauro —
You've loved the wild, untamed me since day one in 2005. You see me — my fire, creativity, and higher self — and have always made space for all of it.
You've always been my soft place to land and the gentlest, safest love I've ever known.
Your consistency grounds me. Your dedication to health inspires me.*

*And your cooking? Truly elite, Legendary, actually.
Thank you for showing up with steady love, for believing in me without hesitation, and for building a life with me that feels nourishing, calm, and full of adventure.
You're the best Dada — and my favorite person to explore this world with.
Love you, Mr. Love Love.*

ACKNOWLEDGMENTS

To my friends and family—

Thank you for riding with me through every wild idea, late-night dream, and creative detour. You've never tried to make me smaller—just louder, brighter, and more myself.

Your humor, quirks, love, and relentless hype have shaped me in the best ways. I am so grateful to be surrounded by such a bold, brilliant, and beautifully original tribe. Thanks for always having my back and for making the journey way more fun.

To my mama—

I chose the perfect mama for this life. You are the *corazón* of our family—resourceful, generous, and fiercely loving. From *el campo* in the Dominican Republic to building a life in a new country, you've uplifted generations with your hands, your home, and your heart. You've welcomed everyone—*everyone*—with home-cooked meals that taste like love, unwavering advocacy, and *cariño* that makes anyone who walks through the door feel like family.

Your eye for style is timeless—vintage, eclectic, and dreamy. You blend creamy textures, lace, ruffles, and bold patterns into unforgettable looks. Who I am and how I show up in the world is shaped by your artistry. La Chula is a published author. *Te quiero mucho*, Mama.

To my readers—

I'm deeply grateful you've taken time out of your busy lives to be present with me on these pages. May you feel seen, supported, and inspired throughout every chapter.

To every mother I've cared for as a nurse—

Your stories, strength, and honesty have stayed with me long after our time together. You've shaped how I listen, show up, and hold space for others during this sacred chapter of life.

To my coworkers and the medical community—

Thank you for the many hats you wear and the quiet moments of humanity we share. Remember to care for yourself as deeply as you care for others. Keep your light burning—stay kind, curious, and ever-evolving.

To future students in the nursing and medical fields—

May you lead with heart, curiosity, and courage. This work will stretch and shape you in ways you can't yet imagine. Stay open, stay grounded, and remember—every interaction is a chance to make someone feel seen, safe, and cared for. That's the real magic.

And finally, to Izabella Xiomara De Leon—

Your talent is nothing short of luminous. Watching you grow from a tiny baby into the radiant artist you are today has been a privilege. Your art gives this book soul. I'm endlessly proud to be your Auntie.

CONTENTS

FOREWORD

Greetings and welcome!

I'm so excited that you have chosen *All Things Postpartum*.

My name is Dr. Shaunte Gray, and I am a board-certified Obstetrician-Gynecologist.

I have spent more than half of my life as an educator, and almost just as long as both a mom and an OB-GYN.

It is no secret that I absolutely love what I do.

Why do I love it so much?

Because as an OB-GYN, I have the privilege of addressing the beautiful complexities that impact our lives as women.

I love the diversity my career brings— from introducing my teenage patients to their anatomy and the changes of puberty, to delivering gender-congruent care, providing preventive care to women of all ages, and celebrating brand-new lives.

I am a very proud physician.

However, my greatest accomplishment in life has been becoming a mother.

Experiencing my own pregnancy and postpartum journey was beautiful, challenging, scary at times — and mostly humbling.

I am so grateful that the knowledge I gained along the way helped me become a better physician and a better person.

And truthfully, I wish I had a resource like this book to help prepare me for all that was to come.

Each of us carries unique experiences that shape who we are and how we move through the world.

Often, we share these experiences to connect, to heal, and to help others navigate their own journeys.

I have had the joy of seeing our beautiful author, Johaira Dilauro, on both sides of care — as a fantastic postpartum nurse and as a mother embracing her own journey.

It has truly been heartwarming to see her fall in love with motherhood.

Johaira is a very talented artist, an empathetic nurse, a proud mother, and now, a brilliant author.

All Things Postpartum is a heartfelt blend of personal experience and educational insight that will help you navigate your own postpartum journey.

She is uplifting, educational, and empowering throughout these pages.

Topics she explores include:

- Setting realistic expectations
- Coping with the unexpected
- Embracing the whirlwind that is motherhood
- Balancing intimacy and self-love

She writes the way she lives — with passion, resilience, boldness, and love.

I am excited for you to dive into *All Things Postpartum* and all the wisdom it holds.

Enjoy!

– Shaunté M. Gray, M.D., M.S.

INTRODUCTION

Jazmine sat in the hospital room, cradling her newborn as sunlight streamed through the window. Her baby had been born just a few days ago, and she was getting ready for discharge. I walked in to check on her, clipboard in hand, expecting a routine interaction. But as I glanced at her, something gave me pause. Her eyes were red-rimmed, and she stared at the bassinet with an expression I couldn't quite place, "Good morning, Jazmine, are you okay?" I asked gently, pausing by her bedside.

She froze, her hand tightening slightly on the blanket wrapped around her baby. For a moment, she didn't respond. Then, almost in a whisper, she said, "Not really."

The words seemed to spill out of her, like she'd been holding them back for days — or longer. She told me how everyone kept saying she should be happy, that she should cherish these fleeting moments with her beautiful, healthy baby. But instead of joy, she felt overwhelmed, angry, and impossibly sad. She described a weight pressing down on her, guilt for not feeling grateful enough, for not loving every second of motherhood the way everyone seemed to expect her to.

"They said to sleep when the baby sleeps," she murmured, a bitter edge to her voice. "But how? When the baby sleeps, my brain is going 100 miles an hour on all the things I need to do. I still have to do laundry when I get home and cook dinner, I am too drained to even move. I don't recognize myself anymore."

Listening to her, I could see how lost she felt. I knew the signs—exhaustion, frustration, guilt, and the unshakable feeling of not being good enough. Postpartum depression wasn't just sadness; it was all-consuming. I listened and reassured her that she wasn't alone, that what she was feeling didn't make her a bad mother. No one had told her it was okay to struggle, to not have it all together. And now, here she was, carrying the weight of it all, convinced there was something wrong with her, that she wasn't cut out for motherhood.

This is it - the essence of the postpartum journey. You might think you know what awaits you at the end of this long tunnel, but trust me when I say you cannot comprehend how overwhelming your emotions after giving birth can be until you are the one cradling your child. Your life has changed fundamentally, yet the world around you continues as if nothing has happened, oblivious to the fact that your entire world has shifted on its axis.

If you've experienced this, know that you're not alone. First and foremost, it's important to understand that this is more common than you know. In fact, over half of women with children experience it. Unfortunately, the stigma surrounding it often keeps the conversation silent. Let's change that.

"Welcome to the world, beautiful humans! I am so happy you are here!" This is my welcome message to all the little babies I have the pleasure of helping transition earth-side. My name is Johaira Michelle DiLauro, and I am so grateful this book has found you. I aspire to educate, comfort, and guide you through one of the most transformational eras of your life.

As a profession, I work as a postpartum nurse at a busy metropolitan hospital in Los Angeles, CA. I am deeply passionate about advocating for women and providing them with genuine connection, empowerment, and education.

I have been dreaming of creating a postpartum book that packs in as much education as possible in a meaningful way, filled with self-care guidance and kindness. So, I am with you, as a human being on planet Earth, aspiring for a more vibrant, kind world. I want to hold space for your fears, anxieties, and unknowns. This book was created with so much love, and I aspire to write more books in the future aimed at bringing you comfort, support, and guidance.

I believe we choose our parents for whatever lessons we are meant to learn in this lifetime. We are all doing the best we can with the tools and mental health we are given. So, I say to you—and I am going to repeat this a lot in this book—you are not alone. We are all, in a way, connected. And if this book made its way to you, then know we are most definitely connected, and there is a group of women out there in the world rooting for you and your tiny humans.

I adore babies and new mothers. I love them so much I work part-time at a hospital as a postpartum nurse. I get to witness, support, and guide new life from hour zero. I take great pride in being an authentic, calming energy as a family transition, welcoming a new member of their household. That's why I decided to write this book. While conversations surrounding the mental impact of childbirth have become more common, there's still a noticeable gap when it comes to discussing how to truly support yourself during those diffi-cult postpartum months. And perhaps even more importantly — to honor that postpartum is not temporary. It marks us, remakes us, and remains with us. We are postpartum — not for a few months, but for the rest of our lives.

In this book, I want to share my knowledge, my experiences, and, most importantly, my heart with you. My goal is to provide a trans-formative perspective on the postpartum journey, focusing on both emotional and physical healing. We'll explore insights from diverse voices and uncover global postpartum practices that offer wisdom and inspiration. This book is meant to walk alongside you, offering guidance, empowerment, and encouragement during this remarkable chapter of your life.

Postpartum can feel overwhelming, but together, we can shift that narrative. I aim to help you see this time not as something to endure, but as an opportunity for strength and growth. Let's reframe this experience as one of transformation and resilience—because you deserve that, and so much more.

But how do we do that? Through honest conversations, self-reflection, and practical tools, we'll navigate the physical and emotional changes that come with postpartum.

First things first, we'll dive into **emotional well-being**—tackling things like anxiety and depression that may come up at some point throughout your journey. Then, we'll talk about **physical recovery,** helping you heal and regain your strength., Plus, we will spend time on self-care and holding onto your sense of identity as you navigate motherhood.

What sets this book apart? It's filled with actionable tools you can start using immediately. Clear communication to simplify complex concepts. Visually stunning art to inspire you with visual pages where you can doodle, write, and express yourself. Thoughtful affirmations and reflection prompts encourage you to pause, breathe, and reconnect with your emotions. Each resource is thoughtfully designed to enhance your life—starting today.

Lastly, I want you to know that you are officially part of a collective of women that honor and support you. You have a community of women who understand what you're going through and are here to empower you every step of the way. This book is for all mothers, of all ages and cultural backgrounds—all of us navigating the beautiful and challenging experience of motherhood. I truly understand the challenges and concerns you're facing. This book addresses them head-on, providing answers and reassurance.

My hope is that this book becomes a guiding light for you, a companion through the ups and downs of postpartum and beyond. Together, we will celebrate the small wins, acknowledge the challenges, and find balance in the chaos of recovery and new motherhood. Postpartum is a unique and transformative journey—one that you don't have to navigate alone. Take a deep breath, trust in your strength, and know that you are taking a delicious massive step in up leveling your personal growth.

This is your space to heal, to learn, and to thrive. Let's go!

CHAPTER 1
THE WILD RIDE OF POSTPARTUM LIFE

When I first began working in postpartum care, I quickly noticed how many new mothers were surrounded by silence and uncertainty. It wasn't the peaceful kind of silence but one filled with unanswered questions and hidden worries. I remember meeting a mother named Sarah, holding her newborn with love but also clear hesitation. "Am I doing this right?" she asked quietly. That question always sticks with me because this woman, who had given her literal flesh and blood to make the baby in her hands, was now looking at me to provide her with some sort of reassurance. That she was doing well, that she was enough.

It breaks my heart to see how much self-doubt and fear can consume a new mother's mind.

The term "fourth trimester" is not just a catchy phrase. Because no matter how much we want to be done with our pregnancy, the reality is that our bodies and minds are still going through a huge transformation. The physical changes may be more apparent, but the emotional and mental changes can often go unnoticed.

That's why understanding the postpartum journey is so crucial. It's not just about healing physically; it's also about navigating the emotional and mental challenges that come with becoming a mother. Think of it this way - your body is healing, your emotions are recalibrating, and your identity is reshaping. This is a crucial time when providing consistent care and nurturing, which is essential for both you and your baby.

Postpartum healing requires a holistic approach to mind, body and soul.

Healing doesn't happen all at once. It comes in two powerful waves.

Physical recovery is one aspect, and it's important to prioritize your physical well-being by taking care of any postpartum complications, following your doctor's recommendations, and practicing self-care. Your uterus, once home to your little one, is now contracting and undergoing involution, gradually returning to its pre-pregnancy size. This process can feel like mild to moderate cramps—some women even describe it as similar to contractions. It's a little reminder of the life your body has nurtured.

But another significant aspect is emotional recovery. This can be a complex and challenging journey, as you navigate through the over-whelming emotions that come with motherhood. Your body is adjusting to its new function as a milk-producing machine, and sleep deprivation can make everything feel more intense. It's perfectly normal to experience a range of emotions during this time, from joy and love to frustration and sadness. Remember that there is no one right way to feel—you are allowed to have conflicting emotions.

As if all of that wasn't enough, you also need to be prepared for the unexpected curveballs that might come your way!

1.1 EXPECTING THE UNEXPECTED

Let me tell you the story of the day my baby was born because I had a dramatic postpartum experience myself. The birth itself was quite beautiful, but immediately after, my placenta wouldn't release on its own, leading to a sudden and severe postpartum hemorrhage. The blood flow was alarmingly heavy—like a river—and it took an entire medical team to help control the situation. Later that night, just as I was trying to process what had happened, I noticed my baby spitting up a large amount of colostrum out of his nose. Panicked and afraid something might be wrong, I called for a NICU doctor to evaluate him. I was devastated when they diagnosed him with a posterior cleft lip and informed me that he would need multiple surgeries, along with additional testing, to rule out other potential complications.

That was just night one.

I cried, mourned, and mentally prepared myself for the battle ahead —because for my baby, I was ready to do anything. Then, by what felt like a miracle, 48 hours later, the diagnosis was reversed. It turned out to be a misdiagnosis, and my baby was perfectly healthy. I left the hospital feeling overwhelmingly grateful to be alive and relieved that my baby was okay. Those 48 hours were so traumatic that I didn't have the time or space to process any of it.

But the trials were far from over.

When I arrived home, it was the peak of a scorching heat wave, and our air conditioner had broken. What followed can only be described as a postpartum crash. Between the hormonal roller coaster of days 3 to 5 postpartum—when pregnancy hormones plummet and milk-producing hormones spike—and all the swelling from IV fluids, blood transfusions, and fluid retention, I felt like I had completely lost control of my body.

It was a legit shit show. Even as someone who worked in the mother-baby world, I was completely unprepared for the sheer chaos of it all.

Here's the thing, though - expecting the unexpected is a skill that every new parent must learn. No matter how much research we do, or how many parenting books we read, there will always be surprises and challenges along the way. It's all part of the journey.

It's important that we don't let these unexpected events consume us. In this new beginning, give yourself permission to embrace imperfection. After all, this isn't just about making it through the postpartum period in one piece—it's about thriving, fueled by knowledge, compassion, and the undeniable fact that you're absolutely crushing it (even if your shirt is covered in spit-up).

1.2 BUCKLE UP FOR THE EMOTIONAL ROLLERCOASTER

Motherhood is often painted as pure bliss, full of endless joy and love. And while there really are an abundance of moments that feel this way, it's not the whole story. A lot of moms find themselves riding a wave of emotions—from pure happiness to intense anxiety. It's totally normal, and a big part of it comes down to the massive hormonal shifts after giving birth. The same hormones that helped grow your baby now have to settle down, and that adjustment can feel like a wild roller coaster ride.

Anxiety is another common part of the mix. It can sneak up on you out of nowhere—you might start second-guessing every little decision or worrying if you're doing things "right." I recall speaking with a mother who shared how she would lie awake at night, anxiously replaying the day's events, wondering if she had made any mistakes. These feelings are normal, but they can become all-consuming and impair everyday life.

Now, let's talk about the "baby blues." If you've never heard of it, let me be the first to tell you—it's real. Those hormonal shifts, the lack of sleep, and the huge responsibility of caring for a newborn can leave you feeling super emotional. Mood swings, random crying, anxiety, irritability—it's all part of the package for many new parents. But here's the thing: feeling this way doesn't mean you're doing anything wrong. Understanding and accepting these emotions is such a huge part of getting through this challenging but oh-so-worth-it journey.

However, this is not the only emotional hurdle that new parents face. Postpartum depression and other mood disorders are also a reality for many individuals.

Studies show that postpartum depression (PPD) affects approximately 1 in 7 women after giving birth, according to the American

Psychological Association. Furthermore, an estimated 10% of fathers also experience symptoms of postpartum depression. That is why it's crucial to be aware of the signs and symptoms and to seek help if needed.

But how do you know it's something more serious? Here are some pointers to look out for:

- Persistent feelings of sadness, hopelessness or despair
- Loss of interest in activities you once enjoyed
- Difficulty bonding with your baby
- Changes in appetite and sleep patterns
- Extreme mood swings and irritability

If you experience any of these symptoms for longer than two weeks, it's important to seek help from a healthcare professional. There is no shame in seeking support during this challenging time. Remember, taking care of yourself is just as important as taking care of your newborn.

1.3 ADJUSTING TO THE NEW NORMAL

Becoming a parent means adjusting to a whole new way of life. I clearly remember mourning my lack of autonomy (doing whatever you want whenever you want). It can be overwhelming and exhausting, but it's important to remember that you are not alone. Many new parents struggle with the demands of parenthood and it's completely normal to feel overwhelmed.

The emotional cost of parenting is something that is often overlooked. The constant worry and pressure to do everything "right" can take a toll on anyone's mental health. That's why it's important to find healthy ways to cope with the stress and challenges of being a new parent.

During my own postpartum journey, I often wanted help with cleaning but felt embarrassed to verbalize it. Sometimes, I'd feel like I needed to tidy up before letting someone else step in—

completely counterproductive, right? So, how do we cope with these emotions?

1. **Don't be afraid to ask for help.**
   - Support from your partner, family, or friends is crucial during postpartum.
   - Remember, it takes a village to raise a child, and asking for assistance doesn't make you any less capable as a parent.
2. **Prioritize self-care.**
   - Incorporate small self-care activities into your routine, even if it's just a few minutes a day.
   - Practices like deep breathing, mindfulness, or meditation can reduce stress and help you feel grounded.
   - Create a calming home environment with soft lighting or soothing music, even if you're working within a small space.
3. **Understand postpartum emotions.**
   - The "baby blues" are common and include mood swings, sadness, and unexplained crying but typically fade after a couple of weeks.
   - If feelings become overwhelming or persist, it could be postpartum depression, and seeking help from a healthcare provider is vital.
   - Journaling can be a helpful outlet for processing your thoughts and emotions.
4. **Set realistic expectations.**
   - Newborns come with unpredictable sleep patterns and feeding challenges.
   - Approach these moments with self-compassion; you and your baby are learning together.
5. **Communicate openly.**
   - Open communication has been a game-changer for me. Sharing my feelings, no matter how small, has lightened my emotional load and made my support network stronger.

- o Try check-ins with your partner or family.
- o Share your feelings, no matter how trivial or embarrassing they may seem.
- o Friends and family often want to help but may not know how—speak up and articulate your needs.

6. **Stay open to new tools.**
   - o Mindfulness and meditation might feel unfamiliar or even overused at first, but they can be powerful tools for staying present and reducing stress.
   - o Even if you're experienced with these practices, there's always room to learn something new.

Postpartum is a blend of challenges and triumphs, and no two stories are the same. Take things one step at a time with patience, support, and self-compassion—you've got this.

1.4 THE BEAUTY OF DIVERSE POSTPARTUM EXPERIENCES

As a Latin-American new mom, Maria struggled to find resources that spoke to her unique needs and cultural background. The continuous spiral of social media comparisons made her feel even more isolated and inadequate. However, the beauty of diverse postpartum experiences is that they are just that: diverse.

So, instead of picturing yourself as the "Martha Stewart" of motherhood, embrace the beauty of diverse postpartum experiences. Every new mom is unique, with her own set of challenges, triumphs, and ways of coping.

And that's perfectly okay.

Letting go of this "perfect mom" ideal can be liberating. I am not saying you won't ever dress up again or can't be a glamorous mama; I am saying it's unrealistic to be that every day. Imagine the freedom of allowing yourself to be human, make mistakes, and grow from them.

Cultural differences also play a significant role in shaping how postpartum emotions are expressed and managed. In some cultures, vulnerability is celebrated as a strength, while in others, discussing feelings openly may be less common. Recognizing and appreciating these differences enriches our understanding of how mothers worldwide cope with postpartum emotions, each in their own unique way.

As a nurse, I have had the privilege of working with new mothers from various cultural backgrounds. One thing that never fails to amaze me is how universal the experience of motherhood is, despite our diverse backgrounds.

Imagine stepping into a home in Malaysia, where a "confinement nanny" guides a mother through the first weeks after birth. This centuries-old practice emphasizes rest, warmth, and nourishment, with healing meals like chicken soup infused with ginger and herbs. These traditions go beyond physical care, embracing a holistic approach to nurture the mother's body, mind, and spirit.

In Korea, new mothers are served "miyeok-guk," a nutrient-rich seaweed soup believed to support milk production and recovery. Similarly, in India, mothers are offered "panjiri," a sweet, energy-boosting mixture of whole wheat flour, nuts, and ghee. These meals are more than sustenance; they are acts of love, crafted to honor a mother's recovery and her role in nurturing new life. Across cultures, food is a vital element of postpartum care, symbolizing the community's support for the mother's well-being. African cultures emphasize the community's shared responsibility in raising the child by performing the "naming ceremony" that honors both the child and the mother.

In many Latino cultures, new mothers often receive hearty soups like "caldo de pollo" (chicken soup), infused with nourishing ingredients such as vegetables, rice, and herbs, believed to promote strength and recovery. These dishes are often prepared by family members, emphasizing the importance of surrounding a mother with love during this vulnerable time.

Similarly, in Jewish culture, the iconic "matzo ball soup" serves as a comforting, restorative meal for postpartum care. For Jewish families, the act of providing this traditional comfort food is a way to reinforce the importance of family and tradition during life's significant transitions.

Meanwhile, in American culture—yes, we do have some—postpartum care might not be steeped in centuries-old traditions, but it's practical. New moms are often supported with gift cards, food delivery services, or organized meal trains from neighbors, friends, and local groups.

These customs—diverse as they may be—share a universal thread: they honor the journey of motherhood.

Diverse Experiences, Shared Resilience

While motherhood is a universal experience, it is deeply personal, shaped by cultural and societal influences. A mother in Sweden may benefit from generous parental leave policies, giving her time to bond with her child without the stress of returning to work too soon. Meanwhile, in Japan, the postpartum period is treated with reverence, with family support woven into the daily rhythm of life. These diverse practices reflect the strength and resilience of mothers across the globe, reminding us of the many paths that lead to the shared goal of nurturing the next generation.

However, societal pressures can complicate the postpartum experience. In many Western cultures, there is a pervasive expectation for mothers to "bounce back" to their pre-pregnancy bodies, often overshadowing the beauty of recovery and transformation. Unrealistic standards of motherhood, perpetuated by media and societal norms, can lead to undue stress and self-doubt. It's vital to remember that every mother's journey is unique, and there is no one-size-fits-all approach to motherhood. Embracing this diversity fosters a more inclusive and supportive environment for all.

For mothers seeking guidance and camaraderie, a wealth of resources is available. Online platforms like Reddit serve as virtual gathering spaces where mothers from all walks of life exchange advice, share stories, and offer encouragement. Subreddits like r/Mommit and r/Parenting foster open discussions about parenting challenges and experiences.

Social media platforms like TikTok, YouTube, and Instagram have also blossomed into vibrant spaces where mothers share their journeys and build supportive communities. You can find additional encouragement, resources, and inspiration by following me on TikTok **@allthingspostpartumbook**. And if my handle ever evolves as our community grows, you can always find me out in the social media world by my name — **Johaira Michelle**.

Specialized support groups and organizations also provide vital assistance. The Black Mamas Matter Alliance offers resources and advocacy for Black maternal health, while Postpartum Support International provides worldwide support for those dealing with postpartum depression and anxiety. La Leche League International is an excellent resource for breastfeeding support, offering both in-person and virtual guidance. Additionally, organizations like Every Mother Counts work to improve maternal care and provide educational resources for mothers globally. These communities and organizations are invaluable, offering expert advice, comfort, and a network of solidarity from those who have walked similar paths.

As we explore the many ways motherhood is celebrated and experienced across cultures, one thing becomes clear: there is no singular definition of what it means to be a mother. By acknowledging and honoring these differences, we gain a deeper appreciation for the strength and beauty inherent in this universal yet deeply personal journey.

1.5 REDEFINING EXPECTATIONS: FROM OVERWHELMING TO EMPOWERING

Do you remember when Amal Clooney gave birth to her twins and was back at work within a few weeks? Or when Beyoncé showed off her incredible post-baby body just months after giving birth to twins? Or even Kate Middleton, who has seemingly mastered the art of effortlessly raising three children while always looking polished and put together?

These are just a few examples of the unrealistic expectations placed on mothers in today's society. The pressure to bounce back quickly after giving birth, to juggle multiple responsibilities with ease, and to maintain a perfect image at all times is immense. These expectations create an overwhelming and often unattainable standard for mothers, leading to feelings of inadequacy, guilt, and self-doubt.

However, it's important to recognize that these women have access to resources and support that most mothers do not. They have nannies, personal trainers, chefs, and other forms of assistance to help them bounce back quickly. For mothers, this is simply not feasible or realistic.

Instead of striving for an unattainable ideal, we should shift our focus towards empowerment. Empowerment often stems from knowledge.

Knowledge is a powerful tool, guiding you through the many decisions that come with motherhood. One thing is to create a vision board and plan for how you want your life to play out, and another thing entirely is to experience all the life lessons along the way. I have been with my husband since the day we met in 2005. I was pretty adamant about not wanting children. I said, "Ask me in 5 years." When 2010 came along, I once again repeated the same phrase.

Something shifted for me in 2011. Although I wasn't ready for babies yet, something inside me felt like I did want to have the experience of being a mother. As I navigated nursing school and really worked on myself as a whole, I realized I had been dealing with anxiety since I was a little girl. I credit so much of my growth as a person to being close to the ocean and truly going deep within to heal.

When I finally became an RN and got my dream job working in a labor and delivery/maternal child health unit, I told my husband, "Okay, I'm ready!" That was November 2017. I ended up having my dream baby in August 2022.

All of that is to say, you never know exactly how your journey to becoming a mother will unfold. Each experience comes with its own trials, life lessons, and stress. I would do it all over again if it meant I got to be a mother, but boy, was this a lesson in perseverance, patience, self-love and kindness.

Holding on to a Sense of Self

Motherhood can feel all-consuming at times, with every aspect of life seemingly intertwined with your new role. But it's important to remember that being a mom is just one part of who you are. Reconnecting with your personal passions and interests can remind you of your individuality and inner strength. Whether it's rediscovering a hobby you love, like painting, or finally diving into that novel on your nightstand, taking time for yourself is essential. Setting personal goals beyond parenting—no matter how small—can feel freeing and energizing. It could be as simple as dedicating time to a creative project or learning something new. These moments are about you, helping you reconnect with the multifaceted person you've always been.

Build That Village

Building a supportive community is another key to thriving as a mom. The saying "it takes a village" exists for a reason. Finding or creating local mom groups, organizing playdates, or even leaning into digital connections can provide valuable support. Sharing experiences, trading advice, and simply knowing you're not alone in this journey can be incredibly reassuring. Social media and online groups also offer opportunities to connect with mothers from all walks of life, providing a platform to share tips, vent frustrations, and celebrate wins — big or small.

As you navigate this new chapter, don't feel tied to a specific formula or path. Redefining your expectations is about creating a life that reflects your values, needs, and desires. Embrace the chaos, celebrate the little victories, and learn from the challenges along the way. Most importantly, remember that becoming a mother doesn't mean losing yourself—it means discovering a new, powerful part of who you are.

Lastly, make choices that bring you peace, and accept that perfection isn't the goal—imperfection is where the magic happens. You're capable, resilient, and never alone. A whole community of moms is out there cheering you on and ready to support you.

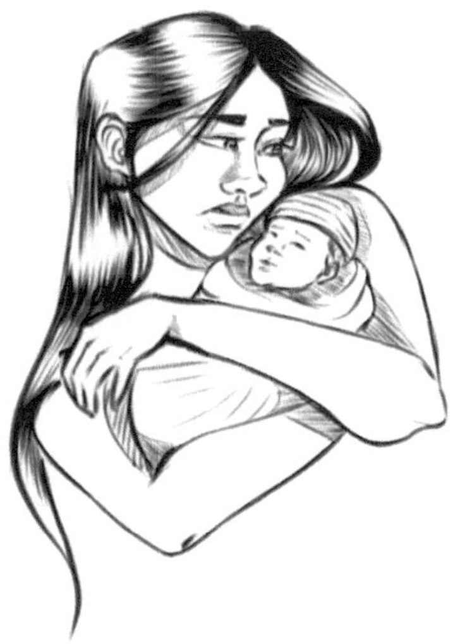

REFLECTION EXERCISE: EMOTIONAL CHECK-IN

As we close this chapter, take a moment to pause and reflect on your emotions. Use this exercise to connect with yourself and process what you're feeling. Here's how to begin:

1. **Choose Your Medium:** Grab a journal, open your phone's notes app, or record a voice or video journal—whatever feels most natural to you.

———————————————————————————————

2. **Ask Yourself:**

• What am I feeling right now?

———————————————————————————————

• What thoughts keep looping in my mind?

———————————————————————————————

• Are there any worries or anxieties that have been lingering?

———————————————————————————————

3. **Let It Out:** As you write, speak, or record, don't judge yourself—just observe. Think of this as "vocal throw up"; let it all out—the good, the bad, and the messy. Be brave and honest. Forget about what anyone else might think—this is your space to be raw and authentic.

———————————————————————————————

———————————————————————————————

4. **End with Self-Love:** After expressing your thoughts, close your reflection with affirmations or a message of self-care. For example:

- Even though I have big feelings, I love and respect myself.
- I am not my thoughts; I am my actions.
- My actions are kind, pure, and enough.
- I love the person I am becoming.
- I am safe, my baby is safe, my family is safe, and we are safe.

This exercise helps you acknowledge your emotions and give them space rather than letting them simmer beneath the surface. Releasing fears and worries has incredible power—it allows us to move forward, lighter and with more clarity.

Remember, this emotional rollercoaster does not define your abilities as a mother or as a person. It's a natural part of growth, and you are not alone. Many others have walked this journey before you, each with their own struggles and triumphs. Give yourself grace, embrace the support around you, and allow yourself to feel everything that arises. This is part of your process, and you are doing beautifully.

CHAPTER 2

MIND MATTERS
KEEPING YOUR SANITY INTACT

As a postpartum nurse, I've had the privilege of witnessing some of the most raw, beautiful, and complex moments of humanity. But one night stands out vividly in my mind. It was just after midnight, and the maternity ward had finally quieted after a long, bustling shift. I was checking on one of my patients, Emily, a first-time mother who had given birth earlier that evening.

When I entered the room, she was sitting upright in bed, cradling her newborn. The baby was asleep, his tiny hand curled around her finger, but Emily's face told a different story. Her eyes were red-rimmed and tired; her brow furrowed as though she was carrying a weight no one else could see. She glanced up at me, startled, as though I had caught her in the middle of something private.

"Hey, Emily," I said softly, not wanting to wake the baby. "How are you feeling?"

She hesitated, her lips parting as if to give the automatic "I'm fine," but then she stopped. Her shoulders sagged, and finally, she said, "I don't know. I should be happy, right? Everyone keeps saying how amazing this is, and how lucky I am. And I know that. I really do. But... I feel so empty. So, disconnected. It's like I'm here, holding him, and I love him, but at the same time, I feel this... dark cloud hanging over me. Like I'm failing already."

Her words poured out in a rush, and I could see the relief on her face from finally voicing what she'd been holding in. I sat down in the chair beside her bed, at her eye level, and offered her a small, reassuring smile. "Emily, it's okay to feel this way," I said gently. "What you're describing sounds a lot like the postpartum blues that can quickly transform into postpartum depression. You've been through something huge – physically, emotionally, mentally. Your hormones are shifting, your body is healing, and you're adjusting to this entirely new role. It's a lot for anyone. Let's get some resources in place. I can reach out to a social worker and provide you with some resources; you don't have to feel all of this alone."

She looked down at her baby, tears sliding down her cheeks. "No one told me it could feel like this," she said, her voice trembling. "All the books, all the stories... They talk about the joy, the milestones, the magic. But not this. Not feeling so... lost."

I remember the blank looks in the eyes of so many mothers when I would ask them how they were doing. The fake smiles, the forced enthusiasm – all masking the reality of what they were feeling. It's like society has this expectation that motherhood should be nothing but pure bliss and fulfillment, and any other emotions are seen as a failure.

My own story with postpartum depression began on day three; when I got home, I went from feeling happy to be home to teary-eyed and angry—like, really, really angry. That hormone drop after pregnancy? I was definitely not prepared for it. I feel like; as a society, we put so much emphasis on labor that we forget the woman and all she experiences after bringing new life into the world.

The trauma of my postpartum hemorrhage lived in my body, but I had no time to process it. Then intrusive thoughts started creeping in throughout the day: *What if I drop this baby? What happens if he's choking and needs me, but I'm here sleeping? I know I have to shower, but what if the blanket goes over his head, and he can't breathe while I'm in the shower?* And the list of dark thoughts went on.

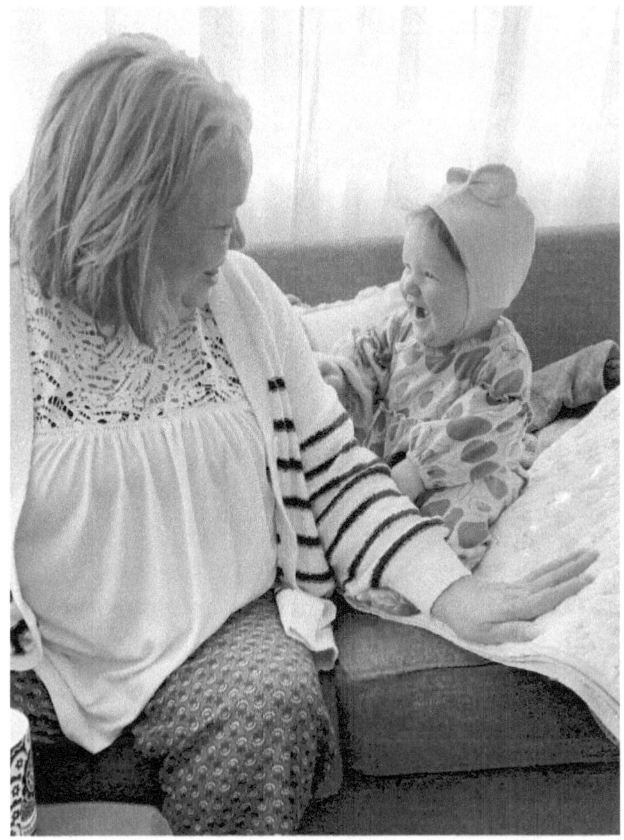

**My mother, Agueda Romero, with my baby, Nikola —
April 14, 2023** Las Vegas, NV | Photo by Johaira Michelle
Dilauro In one of our family's heaviest seasons, Nikola was
the light. The only one who could make my mother smile.

Thankfully, I have been seeing an excellent therapist since 2021. While working as a nurse during the pandemic, I recognized that I wasn't okay. My brother Robert passed away from colon cancer in September 2020. Around the same time, my dad was undergoing dialysis, and my mom suffered a brain aneurysm and stroke in April 2021. The years 2020 and 2021 were challenging. I lost so many people I deeply loved and cherished—Abuela Nenena, Doña Antonia, my nephew Nasser, and Doña Ramona. Grieving in the middle of a global crisis came with its sorrow— gatherings were limited, and the usual rituals of comfort and closure were taken from us.

I felt like I was losing my safety net. I had never experienced loss on this level before. As the healthcare advocate for my family, I carried enormous responsibility and pressure—it was simply too much. I was physically present for everyone, but inside, I was unraveling. It was one of the most challenging seasons of my life—all while trying to conceive and silently fearing that motherhood might never come for me.

This is why it's time to break that stigma. Motherhood is beautiful, yes, but it's also messy, exhausting, and overwhelming at times. And that's completely normal. We need to create a safe space for mothers to share their struggles without fear of judgment or shame. In this chapter, we will discuss the realities of postpartum depression and offer some resources and support for coping with it.

2.1 THE LOWS OF POSTPARTUM DEPRESSION & ANXIETY

You might be familiar with the term "baby blues" – that dip in mood that can come a few days after giving birth. It's completely normal, and is caused by the rapid drop in hormones after pregnancy. But for some women, this feeling doesn't go away after a few days. It lingers and can lead to postpartum depression (PPD).

Postpartum depression is a more profound, more persistent sadness that can linger for months. It often comes with mood swings that feel like storm clouds, unpredictable and heavy. This condition can make even the most minor tasks feel insurmountable and cast a shadow over the experience of bonding with your baby.

Anxiety, on the other hand, can manifest as constant worry or panic attacks, an overwhelming sense of fear that grips you. You may find yourself questioning every decision, consumed by the what-ifs. Both conditions can disrupt sleep and eating patterns, making it hard to find balance.

Certain risk factors can increase the likelihood of experiencing these mental health challenges. These include:

- Personal or family history of depression
- Presence of stressful life events around childbirth (e.g., difficult pregnancy, financial worries)
- Lack of support from partner or network
- Feelings of isolation and being overwhelmed
- Living on Planet Earth at this moment in time

There is no shame in admitting that you are struggling with PPD or postpartum anxiety. It does not make you a bad mother; it does not mean you don't love your baby. These conditions are common and can be treated with therapy, medication, and self-care.

Coping with PPD and Anxiety: Insights, Tools, and Personal Stories

Coping with postpartum depression (PPD) and anxiety can feel overwhelming, but one of the most vital steps in navigating these challenges is self-awareness. Nobody knows you better than you do —not your spouse, your family, or even your closest friends. You are most familiar with your patterns, emotions, and inner thoughts. Developing a deeper understanding of your emotions can help you recognize when something feels off, providing the opportunity to address issues early.

Tracking Your Emotions with a Mood Diary

One practical tool for building self-awareness is a mood diary. By jotting down how you're feeling each day, any significant events, and changes in your behavior or thoughts, you can start to identify patterns and triggers. This simple practice not only prompts daily reflection but also equips you with valuable insights that can be shared with a healthcare provider if needed.

Look for key shifts in your usual behavior, such as finding less joy in activities you once loved, noticing changes in appetite, or struggling to sleep or concentrate. These shifts may indicate it's time to seek help. A structured, daily check-in with yourself can be an essential step in understanding your mental health and taking action when necessary.

Personally, I've found journaling to be extremely helpful in managing PPD and anxiety. But more on that later.

Creating a Positive Environment

Another essential part of managing anxiety is curating the environment around you. I've found that limiting exposure to negativity—whether from TV, music, or social media—has made a significant difference in my life. In 2011, I made the decision to stop watching the news entirely. At first, this was a challenging shift, as I grew up in a household where the news was on constantly. In my childhood, Univision played endlessly in the background with heavy, graphic, and often tragic stories. Looking back, I wonder how much of my intense tantrums as a child were linked to the overstimulation and negativity that I absorbed from having the TV on all the time.

Today, I remind myself that whatever vital information I need will find its way to me. My choice to avoid news and excessive negativity isn't about ignorance—it's about protecting my mental health. I deeply care about the state of the world, but consuming constant negativity caused me immense anxiety and fear, which ultimately benefited no one. Instead, I focus on what good I can do for my family and my community.

This intentionality extends to my professional life as well. As a nurse, I've witnessed how deeply people are attached to external noise, like having the TV or news on for comfort. I've been present in labor rooms where a baby is born, and the news blares in the background. Even during postpartum recovery, the TV often remains on, pulling attention away from one of life's most sacred moments.

When possible, I gently ask families if I can turn the TV down while I provide teaching or encourage them to rest. Sometimes, I'm met with resistance because people are so accustomed to this background noise—it feels "normal" to them. But I believe these moments are worth reclaiming. The birth of a child deserves full presence and connection, free from distractions.

The Role of Technology in Sacred Moments

One of my greatest triggers is seeing how technology dominates our lives, even during life-altering experiences. Over the years, I've noticed a pattern in labor rooms: a baby arrives, the energy is electric and miraculous, and within minutes, family members are on their phones. Some are texting loved ones about the baby's arrival, others are scrolling social media, and a few are making video calls.

While I understand the desire to share the good news right away, it's heartbreaking to see such sacred moments interrupted. I've even incorporated this observation into the maternity tours I lead at my hospital. During these tours, which include educational sessions for expectant parents, I discuss these patterns and encourage families to be mindful of technology's role during these precious moments.

I remind them that the first hours of a baby's life are an incredible time to bond, reflect, and simply be present. While it's natural to want to update friends and family, those messages can wait. The chance to soak in the miracle of life is fleeting, and it's worth focusing on the here and now.

Simple Tools for Emotional Reflection

Simple, reflective tools and exercises can also be incredibly helpful in managing PPD and anxiety. Self-assessment questionnaires or guided questions like "What am I feeling right now?" or "What thoughts are occupying my mind today?" offer structured ways to test your mental state. These tools encourage introspection and can shed light on aspects of your emotional health that might go unnoticed in the busyness of daily life.

Whether you're tracking your mood in a journal, limiting exposure to negativity, or reclaiming sacred moments from the grip of technology, these small steps can have an impact. Coping with PPD and anxiety often involves making intentional changes, both big and small, that prioritize your mental health and well-being.

2.2 BUILDING A MENTAL HEALTH TOOLKIT

Journaling, mindfulness, and creative expression are powerful tools that can transform your mental health, even amidst the chaos of daily life. As a mother, I've leaned on these practices to navigate the highs and lows, finding moments of clarity and calm that anchor me through it all. In this section, I'll share how you can build your own mental health toolkit, starting with simple habits that make a big impact.

The Power of Journaling

When I first started journaling, I was amazed at how this simple act could significantly improve my emotional well-being. Those blank pages became a safe space where I could express my thoughts and feelings without judgment. Journaling isn't just about recording events—it's a therapeutic tool that helps process emotions, reduce stress, and find clarity in this life.

If you're new to journaling, guided prompts can make it easier to get started. One practice I've found great is writing down something you're grateful for, no matter how small. It could be a quiet moment with your baby or the warmth of your morning coffee. Focusing on gratitude shifts your perspective to the positives in life, fostering a sense of balance and grounding.

Mindfulness Practices for Everyday Calm

Mindfulness is another powerful way to support your mental health. Staying present helps reduce anxiety and bring calm, even on the busiest days. One simple mindfulness technique is focused breathing. Whenever you feel overwhelmed, close your eyes, take a deep inhale, hold for a moment, and then exhale slowly. With each breath, imagine the tension leaving your body. This practice has been a lifesaver for me during stressful moments, offering a quick mental reset When my brain is moving too quickly and I am having a hard time going within. I love looking at beautiful flowers, trees, or a view of nature. I become fully present in what I am witnessing. This too is mindfulness.

For a deeper experience, mindful meditation can be transformative. Set aside just a few minutes each day to sit quietly, letting your thoughts come and go without judgment. Another technique I love is the body scan.

Tapping, properly known as emotional freedom technique (EFT), is an all-time favorite of mine. It involves using your fingers to tap on specific acupressure points while making statements about the issue at hand. This helps release any energy blockages and reduce negative emotions or physical discomfort. Tapping can be used during pregnancy, labor, and postpartum to help with anxiety, pain management, and emotional well-being. It can even be used to help with breastfeeding difficulties or baby bonding. This simple technique can provide a sense of control and empowerment during a time when so much feels out of our hands.

Lying down, focus on each part of your body from your toes to the top of your head, releasing tension. This practice not only relaxes the mind but also improves sleep quality—a gift for anyone navigating sleepless nights.

Creative Expression as Emotional Release

Sometimes, words aren't enough to process emotions. That's where creative expression comes in. For me, drawing and doodling have been incredibly freeing. Whether I'm sketching a scene from my day or simply letting my hand move freely, the act of creating helps me release feelings I can't put into words.

Music and dance are also wonderful outlets. On particularly stressful days, I turn up my favorite song and let myself dance freely. It's not about technique or perfection—it's about releasing pent-up energy and transforming it into joy. These spontaneous moments remind me of the happiness that can feel distant amidst the demands of life.

Making It Work in Daily Life

Building a mental health toolkit doesn't require hours of your day. Start small, incorporating these practices into your routine in ways that feel natural. Begin your morning with a few deep breaths and a quick gratitude journaling session. Later, take five minutes to doodle, meditate, or dance. Even brief moments of mindfulness and creativity can add up to a meaningful shift in your emotional well-being. I've found that dedicating just 15–20 minutes a day, broken into small chunks, can make a world of difference.

Involving Your Family

I'm a big advocate for seeking mental health support. It takes courage to ask for help, but no one should have to face their struggles alone. As humans, we thrive in community. While reaching out for professional help may feel unnatural, especially during hard times, it can truly be life-changing.

Even just having someone to listen to and support you can make a huge difference. During my postpartum experience, I wasn't only dealing with intrusive thoughts—I also felt a lot of anger, mostly directed at my husband. Not because he was doing anything wrong, but I think it's easier to feel angry with someone you trust deeply.

That first year postpartum was incredibly challenging for my mental health. I felt so much love and gratitude for my baby and adored watching him grow. But I was also exhausted, overwhelmed, and longing for the family support I didn't have, as we live far from relatives.

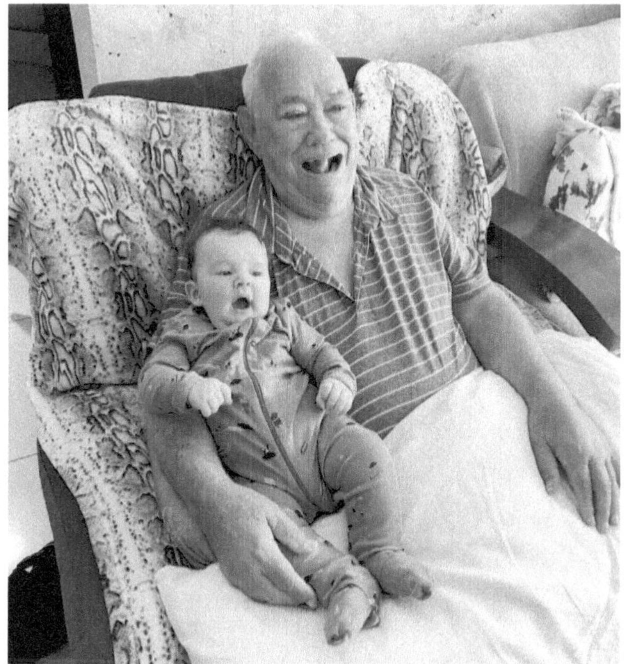

My father, Armando Romero, with his grandson, Nikola — December 18, 2022 Puerto Plata, Dominican Republic | Photo by Johaira Michelle Dilauro Their days together on this earth were short, but the memories are timeless. His dream was to see me become a mother. Mission accomplished.

Things got even harder when my baby was six months old, and my dad—my favorite person in the world, Armando Emmanuel Lizardo Romero—passed away. He was my first love, and I'm so grateful he got to meet his grandson before he left. Losing him was devastating. No matter how expected it may be due to age or illness, losing a parent is heartbreaking. I'm forever grateful to those who supported me during that heavy time.

However, it wasn't easy. I lost two close friendships during this period. Navigating such a profound loss while raising a baby was overwhelming, and feeling misunderstood and judged made it even harder. It was a difficult time, but it taught me the importance of leaning on those who truly understand and support you.

Your mental health journey doesn't have to be a solo endeavor—it can become a shared experience with your family. Talk to your partner or loved ones about your mental health goals and invite them to join you. Meditate together, journal side-by-side, or dance as a family. These shared moments foster connection and understanding while building a stronger support network. Working together as a family creates a sense of unity and strengthens emotional balance.

All of this is to say—it's okay not to be okay. But it's also very necessary to seek help during this time. Be around people who feel like sunshine. The ones who allow you to be authentically you. The ones who love you unconditionally and are there to hold you and support you through heavy and dark times.

Guided Journaling Prompts

If you're looking for inspiration, here are some prompts to enrich your journaling practice:

- What are three things I'm grateful for today?
- How did I navigate a challenging moment today?
- What is one thing I accomplished today?

These prompts encourage self-reflection and help you approach your emotional well-being with mindfulness and intention.

2.3 BOOSTING CONFIDENCE AS A NEW MOM

You know what kills progress? Perfectionism. We all know the voice in our head that says we're not doing enough or we're not good enough. But guess what, mama? You are more than enough exactly as you are, and you are doing an amazing job.

As a new mom, it's too easy to fall into the trap of perfectionism, where each task feels like a test you must ace. But the truth is, there's no perfect way to be a mother. Practicing self-compassion means treating yourself with the kindness and understanding you'd offer a dear friend. It's about forgiving yourself for not having all the answers and recognizing that you are learning and growing.

One technique is to reframe your inner dialogue. Instead of saying, "I messed up," try, "So this is an area of growth" This subtle shift in language can have a powerful impact on your self-image and confidence.

Another favorite of mine is replacing the word should from my vocabulary. I shift with "could." For example, instead of thinking I should be washing the dishes, I say I could wash them, but I am actually going to get in the bath right now.

Affirmations are simple, positive statements that can help reframe our mindset and boost our confidence. Here are some examples:

- I am enough, just as I am.
- I trust myself to make good decisions.
- I embrace imperfection and see it as an opportunity to learn and grow.
- I am strong and resilient
- I nurture my baby with love and patience

These affirmations reinforce your inner strength and remind you of your natural nurturing qualities. Speak them aloud, write them down, or place them where you can see them often. By repeating them regularly, you can start to build a more self-compassionate mindset and strengthen your confidence as a new mom.

2.4 HOLDING SPACE FOR A MAMA WHO IS GRIEVING

To anyone who has ever lost a fetus or a baby—at any stage, for any reason, no matter how much time has passed—I want to hold space for you.

I honor you.
I see you.
I send you love.

One of the most healing books I've ever read is *Spirit Babies* by Walter Makichen. I first heard about it from the magical Kathrin Zenkina, creator of the Manifestation Babe podcast. I had never encountered the concept or language of "spirit babies, " which opened something in me. It brought peace, perspective, and healing that I didn't even know I needed.

Let this be your permission:
To be forever healing.
To continue shedding layers of grief, trauma, and growth.
To redefine yourself again and again in this ever-evolving reality we call motherhood.

2.5 UTILIZING PROFESSIONAL SUPPORT

Yes, you might be doing all the mental work of self-reflection and self-compassion, that doesn't mean you don't need help. And I don't mean the help of a friend or family member, but the help of a trained professional. We are all humans navigating life in a very interesting moment in time. It's brave to seek professional help. Recognizing when to seek professional support is an essential aspect of maintaining your mental health.

When to Seek Professional Support

- When your emotions and mental chatter are interfering with your daily life and, it is affecting your relationships.
- When you feel overwhelmed and unable to cope with your feelings.
- When you experience persistent negative thoughts about harming yourself or others.
- When you have tried a variety of tools and feel you need support to create your own personalized mental health tool kit.

If any of these apply to you, it may be time to seek help from a mental health professional.

How to Seek Professional Support

The process of seeking professional support can seem daunting, but there are steps you can take to make it more manageable:

1. Start by contacting your health insurance provider to see if they cover mental health services and which providers are in-network.
2. Once you have a list of potential therapists, reach out to schedule an initial consultation or phone call to get a feel for their approach and see if it's a good fit for you.
3. Ask for recommendations from friends or family members who have gone through similar struggles.
4. Do some research on therapists or counselors in your area.

Additionally, I highly recommend reaching out to a Social worker. SW are an excellent resource for support groups, community resources and can help you navigate the services available to you.

Finding the right therapist might take a bit of effort, but it's so worth it. Think of it like dating—you might not find the perfect fit right away, and that's okay. Keep trying until you find someone who you feel comfortable opening up to and who can provide the support and guidance you need.

Asking for help is not a sign of defeat or weakness; it takes courage and strength to recognize when you need support. So, don't be afraid to reach out and seek professional help if you feel like you need it. Your mental health is just as important as your physical health, and seeking support can greatly improve your overall well-being.

In this season of your life, seeking professional support is one of the best gifts you can give yourself. It's about acknowledging your needs and ensuring you have what you need to feel whole and supported. Whether it's therapy, a support group, or a hotline, there's help out there for you. Reaching out is a powerful act of self-love, and you deserve every bit of support the world can offer. You are most definitely not alone, even though sometimes it may feel like it. I want to motivate you to seek out resources in your community and choose to believe there are brighter, more balanced days ahead.

As we reach the end of this chapter, remember that boosting your confidence as a new mom is a continuous, evolving process. It's about embracing self-compassion, celebrating your achievements, and finding joy in the connections you make. These practices are not just about surviving motherhood but thriving within it and finding empowerment in everyday moments. My wish for you is to be held, loved, and pampered during this moment in time. You are worthy of love. You deserve to feel safe and cared for.

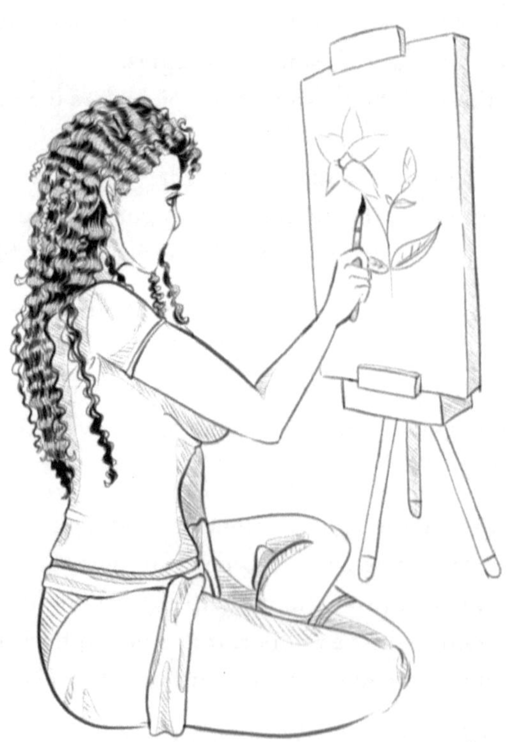

Exercise for Reflective Self-Assessment

Take a moment to complete this brief self-assessment to reflect on your emotional well-being:

1. Have I noticed any changes in my mood or energy levels recently?

____

2. Am I finding it challenging to bond with my baby?

____

3. Have my sleeping or eating habits changed in any way?

____

4. Am I experiencing any physical symptoms such as headaches, stomachaches, or muscle tension?

____

5. Have I been able to find time for self-care and activities that bring me joy?

____

6. Do I feel supported by my partner, family, and friends in my role as a new mom?

7. Do I have someone I can talk to about my feelings and concerns without judgment?

8. Have I reached out for professional support if needed?

9. Overall, how satisfied am I with my emotional well-being at this moment in time?

Use these questions to check in with yourself regularly. Reflect on your answers and consider how they might impact your overall mental health.

Action Step:

If you notice concerning patterns or feel overwhelmed, take the brave step of seeking support.

CHAPTER 3

BOUNCING BACK LIKE A PRO

THE DELIVERY & RECUPERATION

Becoming a mother is a journey like no other. You can read all the books, take all the classes, and ask every woman you know about their experiences—but nothing can truly prepare you for the moment you bring a human being into the world. Katalina, a first-time mom, shared her story. "The delivery went smoothly, but I wasn't prepared for what came after. I thought postpartum healing would just mean a bit of rest, but I felt like my body was a stranger. Walking hurts, sitting hurts—heck, even laughing hurts. I'd look in the mirror and wonder, 'Will I ever feel like myself again?'"

Emily, another mom, added her voice to this shared reality. "I knew my body would change, but I didn't expect to feel so alien in my own skin. It was like waking up in a body that didn't belong to me anymore."

For so many mothers, the postpartum phase is a surprising mix of awe and frustration. The body, having performed the miracle of childbirth, often struggles with the aftermath—aches, exhaustion, and unfamiliarity. These profound physical changes can be accompanied by added stressors that slow the healing process. But here's the thing: healing takes time, patience, and care.

Motherhood is a transition—not just emotionally but physically. It's a reminder of the incredible resilience of the human body and the importance of giving it the grace it deserves. For new moms, this phase may feel foreign and even overwhelming, but it's also a testament to their strength. While it's not an easy road, it's one worth walking, knowing that every day brings a little more familiarity and strength.

The physical toll that this transition takes on a mother's body can be staggering. And I'm not telling you this to scare you, or to make you relive the trauma your body went through. But rather, to remind you that it's okay not to feel like yourself in the months after giving birth. It's okay to focus on your own physical healing alongside caring for your baby.

3.1 MY POSTPARTUM JOURNEY: A PERSONAL STORY

Quick synopsis of my birth story: 41 weeks and 3 days, from planning to birth at home to being induced to having a postpartum hemorrhage.

Even though getting pregnant was not a smooth process for me, being pregnant was awesome. I loved it so much. I felt strong, beautiful, and motivated to complete absolutely everything I had ever dreamed of in record time. I was in film school while working at the hospital. I worked as a producer on a short film, and worked on my song and music video for "Rona." Your girl was busy—running around to film festivals, starring in a music video at 40 weeks pregnant—I can genuinely say that during my pregnancy, I was thriving. I was also preparing for what I envisioned to be the dream labor situation. I practiced my hypnobirthing modules, squatted for extended amounts of time, and kept myself active and healthy.

Meanwhile, the baby was showing zero signs of wanting to be born. I think he was having too much fun turning up in my belly and soaking up all the love being poured onto us. I even decided to rent a pregnancy tub so that I could labor at home and then arrive at the hospital when I was 7-8 cm dilated.

I was 41 weeks and 3 days pregnant, going on 5-mile hikes, dancing, grooving, and envisioning my labor. At this point, my relaxed demeanor turned into worry. "Let's go get induced," I said, all relaxed at the farmer's market while eating a breakfast sandwich with my mom and husband.

So, I went to the hospital, still holding on to a plan for how I wanted my labor to go. Once they started Pitocin and artificially broke my water, things got real FAST. Five hours into a howling-at-my-ancestors labor, I tapped out and said, "Knock me out." Meaning, yes to the epidural. Once I had some pain relief, the labor went rather smoothly. Fifteen minutes of pushing—my personal favorite part of labor—and there I was, catching my slippery baby onto my chest. We did it. Five years of manifesting, praying, meditating, and surrendering.

Twenty minutes later, in what felt like forever, I experienced a postpartum hemorrhage where I lost 3.6 liters of blood. Things got scary fast. Luckily, I had a dream team, and all hands were on deck. After several blood transfusions and many medications, I was stable. Three days later, I was home.

3.2 WHAT TO EXPECT IMMEDIATELY AFTER DELIVERY

Understanding Postpartum Hemorrhage: The Leading Cause of Maternal Mortality

Your birthing experience may have gone smoothly, but sometimes complications can arise after giving birth that requires a blood transfusion. This is when blood from a donor is given to someone who needs it due to severe bleeding or other medical conditions. Postpartum hemorrhage, which is defined as losing more than 500 ml of blood for vaginal delivery and 1000 ml of blood for c-section delivery, within the first 24 hours, is one of the main reasons for blood transfusions. There are various procedures and medications that are used to stop a postpartum hemorrhage, but if the blood loss causes significant anemia, then a blood transfusion is indicated. There are a variety of factors that increase the risk of postpartum hemorrhage, but some common ones are pre-existing anemia, long labors, large babies, and placental problems.

Anemia during pregnancy is one of the most preventable conditions —and the good news is, prevention can start right on your plate. Eating an iron-rich diet and taking iron supplements, if recommended, can make a big difference. A helpful tip: pair iron-rich foods with those high in vitamin C to increase absorption. Some of my personal favorites include dried fruits, dark leafy greens like spinach, and all kinds of beans—black beans, lentils, navy beans, pinto, and black-eyed peas (shout out to all the beans!). You'll also find iron in fortified foods like pasta and breads. Pairing them with vitamin C-rich options—like citrus fruits, berries, broccoli, or broccolini—can help your body absorb iron more effectively.

If anemia does occur and becomes severe, a blood transfusion may be recommended. While the idea of receiving someone else's blood can feel intimidating, it's reassuring to know that all blood is thoroughly screened and tested for safety. Transfusions can be life-saving and play a key role in recovery, especially after childbirth. Always feel empowered to ask questions and stay informed about your care —you deserve to understand your body and your options.

Warning signs to watch for after giving birth include excessive bleeding, dizziness, and fatigue. Seeking immediate medical care is crucial if you experience these symptoms, as postpartum hemorrhage can rapidly become a serious and life-threatening condition.

Recognizing and Managing Preeclampsia

You know how every time you went for prenatal visits; your blood pressure was measured? It wasn't just a routine check—it helps monitor your health and identify conditions like preeclampsia and gestational hypertension (a precursor to preeclampsia). Even though we don't yet fully understand what causes it, preeclampsia can quickly develop into a severe condition which can cause liver damage, kidney damage, and seizures. Preeclampsia typically develops later in pregnancy and is characterized by high blood pressure that arises after 20 weeks. It is often accompanied by signs of issues with the kidneys, liver, or central nervous system. Common symptoms include headaches, blurred vision, and upper abdominal pain. While swelling of the hands and feet is common, widespread body swelling is another indicator of preeclampsia, usually appearing in more advanced stages of the condition. These symptoms can also be caused by other conditions, making it challenging to determine if it's truly preeclampsia. It's important to have your blood pressure checked if you experience any of these symptoms. . For most people, preeclampsia is cured when the pregnancy is over, but there is still some risk of developing it after childbirth.

Recovery involves closely monitoring your blood pressure, possibly taking medications, and giving your body the rest and care it needs. It's a cautious game of balance: staying hydrated, eating well, and not overdoing it. While preeclampsia may take some time to resolve, your body will gradually regain its balance with proper care and support, allowing you to focus on healing and recovery.

As you navigate this recovery process, it's also important to stay vigilant for any signs that might indicate complications.

While many postpartum symptoms are typical, some signs warrant medical attention. Excessive bleeding, large blood clots, severe headache, or signs of infection such as fever or foul-smelling discharge should prompt a call to your healthcare provider. If something feels off, it's always better to seek advice.

Your Changing Body: The First 24 Hours

Uterine involution: How your uterus begins to shrink

Postpartum recovery is full of incredible changes, including the uterus shrinking back to its pre-pregnancy size—a process called uterine involution. This happens through contractions that can feel like menstrual cramps, especially during those first few days after childbirth. If you're breastfeeding, you might notice these "after-pains" are more intense, thanks to the release of oxytocin. While they can be uncomfortable, these sensations are a powerful sign that your body is healing and doing exactly what it's supposed to.

However, it's important to pay attention to the severity and duration of these cramps. If the pain suddenly increases instead of staying stable or decreasing, it may be a sign of an infection or complication. In this case, it's crucial to contact your healthcare provider or return to the hospital for further evaluation.

Additionally, uterine involution is accompanied by postpartum bleeding, known as lochia. This is the shedding of the uterine lining and can last up to six weeks after giving birth. During this time, it's important to use only sanitary pads, as tampons are not suitable for postpartum bleeding. Tampons should be reserved for when your regular period resumes, but for lochia, stick to pads. Again, if you experience heavy bleeding (soaking a pad in one hour) or notice any unusual discharge, don't hesitate to reach out to your healthcare provider.

In Case of Surgery

Once your baby arrives and the surgery is complete, you'll spend a few hours in a recovery room. During this time, medical staff will closely monitor your vital signs to make sure everything is stable. You'll likely have a urinary catheter temporarily and be given pain medication to ease discomfort.

As soon as you feel ready, skin-to-skin contact and breastfeeding can usually start right away. These moments are beneficial for both you and your baby. Don't be afraid to ask for support if you need help getting into a comfortable position for these first precious moments.

Caring for Your Incision

Your incision will need some extra attention as it heals. Keep the area clean and dry, and follow your healthcare provider's instructions carefully. Don't forget to drink water, eat fiber-rich foods, and use stool softeners to avoid straining during bowel movements.

For now, avoid lifting heavy objects or doing anything too strenuous —your body needs at least six weeks to recover before tackling those kinds of tasks.

Managing Pain

Pain is part of the healing process, but it doesn't have to be unbearable. Your doctor might prescribe medication or recommend over-the-counter options, so use them as directed to stay comfortable.

3.3 PAIN MANAGEMENT AND HEALING STRATEGIES

Managing Pain and Discomfort

Postpartum recovery often comes with aches and pains, but there are simple ways to ease them. Cold packs can be a lifesaver for reducing swelling and soothing sore areas like engorged breasts or the perineal region. Keep a few in the freezer, wrapped in soft cloths, and apply as needed for quick relief. Taking prescription pain medication around the clock is very important. If taken correctly, pain can be managed, and you are very unlikely to need narcotic pain medication, even if you had a c-section. It's best to take the prescription ibuprofen and acetaminophen not just when the pain gets strong, but every six or eight hours per the prescription for about a week to keep the pain under control. These medications have cumulative effects, so each dose works better because of the previous dose. Do not wait until the pain gets too strong; take it preventively.

Heat therapy can also work wonders. Whether you use an electric heating pad, a microwavable option, or a classic hot water bottle, the warmth can help ease cramps and discomfort. A warm compress is particularly soothing and can provide instant relief during those tougher moments.

Over-the-counter pain relievers, like ibuprofen or acetaminophen, are safe options (when you are not taking prescription strength) for breastfeeding and can help with both inflammation and pain.

Natural Healing Techniques

For a more holistic approach, natural remedies can complement conventional methods. Herbal teas like chamomile are calming, while ginger is invigorating and can help reduce inflammation. Aromatherapy is another soothing option. Essential oils like rose, geranium, peppermint, or eucalyptus can transform your space into a relaxation haven.

Rest is essential for postpartum recovery, even if it feels nearly impossible with a newborn. Creating a relaxing environment can make a big difference. Dim the lights, play soft music or white noise, and unplug from screens when you can. These small changes signal your body that it's time to unwind.

Speaking of baths, a soak with Epsom salts can be incredibly rejuvenating. The magnesium in the salts helps relax muscles, ease soreness, and turn your bath into a mini spa experience. Sitz baths with Epsom salts are also a great way to soothe discomfort and promote healing for specific areas of the body.

Finding the right sleep position also helps. Use pillows to support your back or legs—whatever feels most comfortable. And remember, sleep when the baby sleeps, even if it's just a quick nap. Let go of the to-do list and prioritize your rest whenever possible. Even short moments of downtime can be restorative.

Supportive garments can make a difference in the postpartum period, but it's important to choose what truly brings you comfort. While some people use postpartum wraps or binders hoping they'll speed up healing, there's no solid evidence that they actually improve recovery. Instead, they can provide gentle compression to support your abdominal muscles, reduce swelling, and offer stability if it feels good for you. Nursing bras, however, are a must-have, delivering comfort and support for changing breasts.

When it comes to clothing, prioritize comfort. Choose soft, stretchy materials that move with you and adapt to your body's needs during this time.

Postpartum recovery is a time to slow down, listen to your body, and give yourself grace. Whether you're soothing aches with a heating pad, sipping on a calming tea, or sneaking in a quick nap, every small act of care makes a difference. Healing takes time—be patient with yourself and embrace this new chapter with as much kindness as you give to your little one.

How to Create Your Postpartum Comfort Kit

Your healing deserves to be honored with care and tenderness.

Create a comfort kit to wrap yourself in support when you need it most:

- **Collect soothing essentials** like cold packs, herbal teas, and calming essential oils.
- **Include gentle pain relief**—whether that's over-the-counter medication, a prescription, or natural remedies.
- **Add layers of coziness** with a soft blanket, a warm robe, or your favorite pair of slippers.
- **Personalize with love**, adding anything that feels nourishing to your spirit—perhaps a favorite book, journal, or a beloved snack.

Once your kit is complete, keep it somewhere you have easy access to. It's your reminder that even in the hardest moments, you are worthy of rest, comfort, and deep care.

3.4 THE FIRST 4-6 WEEKS: HEALING AND ADJUSTING

Many women notice substantial improvement within six weeks, though complete recovery may take more time. Be patient with yourself and attend all follow-up appointments to ensure everything is healing as it should. Remember, everyone's recovery timeline is different, so don't compare your progress to anyone else's.

Navigating Postpartum Urinary Changes

The postpartum period brings incredible changes to your body, especially in your pelvic floor—the muscles of the pelvis that support your uterus, bladder, and rectum, as well as your baby throughout pregnancy and birth. After months of carrying a baby and the act of childbirth itself, these muscles can feel strained or weakened. It's completely normal to experience bladder control issues initially. As a nurse, I've seen countless new moms surprised or embarrassed when they leak a little (or a lot!) in the hospital. The swelling, numbness, and lack of control can feel overwhelming, but let me reassure you: you're not alone, and this is temporary.

Your body just accomplished something extraordinary, and recovery takes time. In those early weeks, your pelvic floor needs rest and healing before you think about strengthening. When you're ready, gentle strategies to retrain and strengthen your pelvic floor can help you regain control and confidence. Begin with basic bladder training: schedule bathroom visits every 2-3 hours, even if you don't feel the urge. This supports your body in finding its rhythm again and prevents an overfull bladder.

As you progress in your recovery, working with a pelvic floor physical therapist can make a big difference. They'll guide you through exercises tailored to your specific needs, focusing on more than just quick muscle contractions. These exercises target the entire pelvic region to rebuild function and strength gradually and effectively. Remember, it's about more than squeezing—it's about reconnecting with your body and giving it the care, it deserves.

If things aren't improving after three months, reach out to your OBGYN or midwife to explore therapy options. There are so many tools and treatments available today to support your healing journey.

Postpartum Depression: Recognizing the Signs and Symptoms

Postpartum depression can manifest in a variety of ways, from persistent sadness and anxiety to difficulty bonding with your baby.

It's important to recognize these signs early so you can seek the support you need.

How and When to Seek Help

If you're feeling overwhelmed or struggling emotionally, don't hesitate to reach out to a trusted healthcare provider. Therapy, support groups, or medication can play a role in helping you navigate this challenging time.

Hormonal Shifts and Their Emotional Impact

Hormonal shifts after childbirth can feel like a second puberty, bringing unexpected physical and emotional changes. For instance, you may notice increased hair shedding—a natural response as your body adjusts from the pregnancy-boosted hair growth phase. While finding clumps of hair in your brush may be unsettling, rest assured it's temporary. Similarly, your skin might feel drier or more sensitive as hormonal fluctuations recalibrate your body back to its pre-pregnancy state.

Hormone Fluctuation and Physical Changes

Postpartum metabolism and weight retention are common concerns. You might even notice swelling after childbirth, which can feel surprising. However, as long as the swelling is evenly distributed, it's nothing to worry about. Most of the time, noticeable improvement occurs by two weeks postpartum.

These hormonal changes also affect energy levels and appetite. You might feel unusually hungry—or not hungry at all—and both are perfectly normal. With so much societal pressure to "bounce back" quickly, it's crucial to remember that your body needs time to heal. Focus on eating a balanced diet, staying hydrated, and giving yourself grace during this period of adjustment.

Emotional Well-Being Tips for New Mothers

- Prioritize rest whenever possible
- Ask for help; this is a time when help is needed and appreciated.
- Take short walks or spend time outside to boost your mood.
- Be patient with yourself—parenthood is a journey, and it's okay not to have all the answers right away.

Your postpartum journey is unique, and it's important to give yourself the time and kindness you deserve to heal and adjust.

3.5 BREASTFEEDING AND EMBRACING POSTPARTUM CHANGES

Breastfeeding can come with its fair share of challenges, and one of the most common is breast engorgement.

As a postpartum nurse, I see moms navigate this often—whether they're breastfeeding or not. Breast engorgement occurs when your breasts become swollen, tender, and overly full. For breastfeeding moms, it's typically a sign of increased milk production as your body adjusts to its new role. However, it's not always a comfortable process. Your breasts may feel hard, sore, and even like they could burst.

For moms who aren't breastfeeding, engorgement can still happen and be just as uncomfortable. Although this feeling and experience flat-out sucks, there are ways to find relief.

Cold compresses or ice packs can work wonders to reduce swelling. Gentle breast massages before and during feedings help stimulate milk flow and ease pressure. If your baby is having trouble latching, consider hand expressing or using a breast pump for a few minutes. Wearing a supportive, well-fitted bra can also help provide comfort without being restrictive.

If discomfort persists, try using warm compresses or taking a warm shower before feeding to help relax the milk ducts and ease the process. However, if you notice a fever, it's important to seek medical advice right away, as engorgement can sometimes lead to mastitis, which may need antibiotic treatment. Keep in mind, this phase is temporary, and your body is doing amazing work to provide for your baby.

A little extra self-care—whether it's icing, massaging, or simply taking a moment to breathe—can make a big difference. Take care of yourself because there will be bumps and hiccups along the way as you transition to this new chapter with your newborn.

3.6 THERE WILL BE CHANGES: STRETCH MARKS AND BODY IMAGE

Stretch marks are like the badges of honor etched into the skin of many mothers. These silvery lines, often seen on the abdomen, hips, and breasts, are a testament to the incredible work your body has done. They are as common as they are varied, with some women seeing them fade over time and others finding them a permanent fixture. Yet, no matter their appearance, stretch marks tell your story. In their candid conversations with me, many mothers have described a sense of surprise and eventual acceptance upon first encountering these marks. "At first, I thought they were battle scars," one mother told me, "but now I see them as part of the beautiful narrative of motherhood." This shift from viewing them as imperfections to embracing them as symbols of strength is a journey worth celebrating.

There's no denying that our bodies will change, but caring for your skin is an act of self-love. Moisturizing creams and oils can help keep your skin supple and may aid in minimizing the appearance of stretch marks. Applying cocoa butter, shea butter, and vitamin E oil regularly, particularly after a warm shower when your skin is most receptive, can make a difference. Using a soft brush or scrub, gentle exfoliation can also promote skin renewal by removing dead cells. It's a simple ritual that nourishes your skin and provides a moment of mindfulness amidst the busy days of motherhood.

The psychological impact of body changes can be extreme, involving self-esteem and body image. Many women find themselves grappling with societal expectations, feeling pressured to "bounce back" to their pre-pregnancy bodies. And very rarely is any woman left out of experiencing body dysmorphia

This pressure can lead to a cycle of negative self-talk and comparison with unrealistic standards often perpetuated by the media. It's vital to break this cycle with mindful self-talk and affirmations. Remind yourself daily of the amazing feats your body has accomplished. Stand in front of the mirror and say:

My body is strong; my body is beautiful.
I honor, love, and respect my body.
I am grateful for all my body does for me.
I am strong, and my body can do amazing things.

These affirmations, though simple, can drastically shift your mindset from criticism to appreciation.

In the face of these challenges, self-acceptance and self-love are essential. Exploring social media hashtags like #BodyPositivity or #PostpartumJourney or engaging with online communities such as The Honest Body Project or Birth Without Fear, can provide a supportive space to share experiences and connect with others. These initiatives celebrate diverse bodies and encourage authenticity, helping you embrace the beauty of every stage of your postpartum journey.

Fashion, too, can be a powerful tool for self-expression. Dressing in clothes that make you feel good, rather than focusing on size or trends, can enhance your confidence. Whether it's a flowy dress that feels like a hug or a pair of pants that fit just right, choose pieces that reflect your personality and comfort.

Be kind to yourself. There is no benefit in belittling yourself or talking down on your evolved body. Speak kindness and gratitude into your body. It is so brave to speak love into your body.

Your body has undergone an extraordinary transformation and deserves to be honored, not hidden. Each mark and curve is a chapter in the story of bringing life into the world. Stand tall in the knowledge that you are part of a long lineage of women who have walked this path, each with their own stories of strength and resilience.

A Message of Resilience

My journey through postpartum hemorrhage and blood transfusion was one of the most challenging experiences of my life. Yet, it also showed me the depth of my strength and the power of a supportive community. For mothers facing similar challenges, know this: you are not alone, and your journey is one of incredible courage. Whether it takes weeks or months, healing is possible, and there is no timeline for reclaiming your sense of self after such a life-changing event.

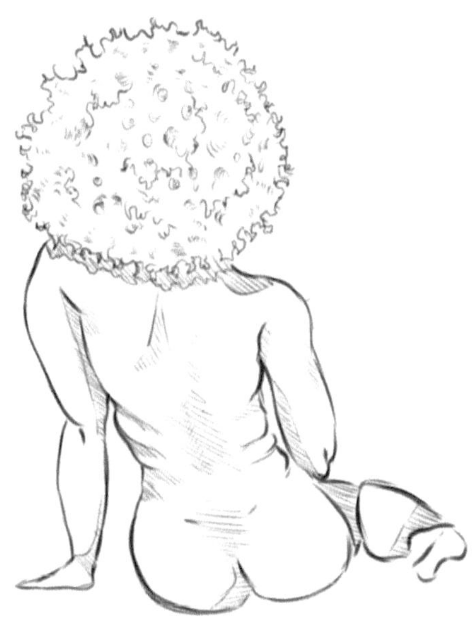

POSTPARTUM BODY SCAN AND RECOVERY EXERCISE

Take a moment to tune in to your body and mind with this gentle recovery exercise. This practice is designed to help you track your healing journey and reconnect with your body as it recovers. You can also keep a journal to note how you feel before and after the exercise or jot down any symptoms, questions, or concerns to bring to your follow-up appointments.

Step 1: Breathing and Gratitude for Your Womb

- Place your hand on your stomach.
- Close your eyes and take five deep, long breaths.
- With each inhale, visualize breathing in bright, sparkly light into your womb, thanking it for all it has done for you.
- With each exhale, whisper "thank you" to your womb, your baby's first home.

Step 2: Head and Brain Relaxation

- Focus on the crown of your head. Imagine a bright, sparkly light shining there.
- Exhale and release all exhaustion, pain, and worry.
- Whisper "thank you" to your brain for managing hormone fluctuations and helping you navigate this journey.

Step 3: Connecting to Your Intuition

- Focus on the space between your eyebrows, your third eye.
- Move this area gently and take a deep breath.
- Thank your intuition for guiding you, and remind yourself that you will seek help when needed.

Step 4: Releasing Through the Throat

- Picture a sparkly light swirling around your throat.
- Take a deep breath, and on the exhale, make an ocean-like sound by constricting your throat slightly.
- Do these five times, imagining the energy of the ocean clearing anything unsaid. Reclaim your voice and power.

Step 5: Shoulders and Neck Release

- Gently sway your head from side to side and take five deep breaths.
- Roll your shoulders and drop them, releasing tension and the weight you've been carrying.

Step 6: Gratitude for Your Breasts

- Place your hands on your chest or gently over your breasts.
- Thank them for all the changes they've undergone, and honor your unique journey, whether you're breastfeeding or not.

Step 7: Digestive Organ Healing

- Breathe deeply into your stomach and digestive organs.
- Imagine bright light energizing this area, thanking your body for its automatic processes.
- Remind your body that it is safe and healing.

Step 8: Full-Body Light Visualization

- Envision a bright light starting at the top of your head and moving down to your hips.
- Picture the light embracing your bladder, ovaries, uterus, vagina, and rectum. Thank these organs for their work and remind them they are healing.

- Let the light flow down your legs, to your ankles, and finally to your toes.
- Wiggle your toes, stretch your feet, and give thanks for your body's strength and resilience.

Step 9: Affirmations

Repeat these affirmations aloud or in your mind:

Thank you, physical body, for providing me with so much strength.
Thank you for healing at the perfect time for me.
My body is safe to heal.
I am safe to heal.
Thank you for sustaining me and my baby.
I promise to nourish you so we can heal together.
I am in the process of healing.

Step 10: Close with Deep Breathing

- Take three deep breaths to end the exercise.
- Feel free to return to this body scan exercise whenever you need to reground yourself.

Gentle Physical Activity (Optional Addition)

When you're ready, ease into gentle movements to support your recovery. Try light yoga stretches, swaying, or simple poses while focusing on relaxation and breathing. Listen to your body, and let this reintegration into movement be gradual and mindful.

CHAPTER 4

MILK, MEALS, AND MOTHERHOOD MAGIC

During one of my shifts, I met Caroline, a new mother cradling her tiny newborn with a mix of exhaustion and uncertainty etched on her face. She hesitated before saying, "I just don't know if I'm doing enough. What if I don't have enough? What if I can't give him what he needs?" Her words struck a very familiar chord—almost every shift I work I hear this concern. Anxiety is shared by so many mothers who worry about providing the best start for their baby, especially when it comes to breastfeeding.

Breastfeeding, often described as a natural act, can feel anything but easy at first. Many mothers, like Caroline, face challenges that leave them questioning their abilities: Will my baby latch properly? Am I producing enough milk? Am I doing this right? These questions aren't born from a lack of care—quite the opposite. They stem from the immense love and responsibility mothers feel, paired with the pressure to meet an ideal that can sometimes seem unattainable.

This is natural. Breastfeeding isn't about perfection; it's about connection. It's about nurturing your baby while also finding a rhythm that works for both of you. From the incredible benefits of colostrum, often called "liquid gold," to tips for navigating common challenges, we'll explore how breastfeeding supports your baby's health and strengthens your bond. And if things don't go as planned, remember this: you are doing enough, and the energy that you give is what truly matters most. Let's dive in and break down the breast-feeding journey—step by step, with support and understanding.

4.1 THE WONDER THAT IS BREAST MILK

Breast Milk is often called a "miracle food" for good reason. It's not just a source of nutrition for your baby but also contains a variety of components that support their health and development. In fact, one drop of breastmilk contains an estimated 1 million white blood cells, which help prevent infections. Here's a closer look at what makes each drop so extraordinary:

Nutrients:

- **Carbohydrates**: Primarily lactose, which provides energy and supports brain development.
- **Fats**: Including essential fatty acids like DHA and ARA for brain and vision development.
- **Proteins**: A combination of whey and casein, providing building blocks for growth and easy digestion.
- **Vitamins and Minerals**: Including calcium, magnesium, potassium, zinc, and vitamins A, D, E, and K to support bone development and growth.

Immune-Boosting Components:

- **Antibodies (Immunoglobulins)**: Protect the baby against infections and strengthen the immune system.
- **White Blood Cells**: Actively fight pathogens and protect against illnesses.
- **Lactoferrin**: Inhibits the growth of harmful bacteria and enhances iron absorption.
- **Oligosaccharides**: Feed beneficial gut bacteria and prevent the growth of harmful microbes.

Hormones and Growth Factors:

- **Epidermal Growth Factor (EGF):** Promotes the development of the gut lining.
- **Adiponectin and Leptin:** Regulate appetite and metabolism.
- **Stem Cells:** Support tissue repair and development.

Enzymes and Bioactive Compounds:

- **Lipase:** Helps break down fats for easier digestion.
- **Amylase:** Aids in carbohydrate digestion.
- **Nucleotides:** Support immune function and promote healthy cell development.

Dynamic Adaptation: Breastmilk is not static; its composition changes:

- **Over Time:** To meet the baby's nutritional needs at different stages.
- **During a Feeding,** Foremilk quenches thirst while Hindmilk provides energy and satiety.
- **In Response to Illness:** When a baby is sick, breast milk increases immune cells and antibodies to fight the infection.

Colostrum: The First Milk

Colostrum, often called "liquid gold," has a fascinating history. Long ago, it was known as the first milk, but people didn't always understand how important it was. In some ancient cultures, it was seen as sacred and essential for newborns, while in others, it was misunderstood or even thrown away because of its thick, yellow appearance. Over time, midwives and healers noticed how much it helped babies thrive and started encouraging its use in some communities.

Fast forward to the late 19th and early 20th centuries, when scientists began digging deeper into colostrum's benefits. It's rich in immunoglobulins and filled with vital nutrients, growth hormones, and antimicrobial properties. In essence, colostrum is a nutritional powerhouse designed to protect and support newborns.

By the mid-20th century, colostrum was finally getting the recognition it deserved as an irreplaceable part of early infant nutrition. Today, its benefits are well-known, from boosting immunity and supporting gut health to promoting overall growth.

It is made during pregnancy and the first few days after birth. Compared to mature breast milk, it is thicker and packed with more nutrients.

Why It's Important: This slow-flow milk is easy for newborns to digest, making it the perfect supplement until your regular supply kicks in.

Nutritional Properties:

- Rich in **antibodies**, particularly IgA, protect the baby's gut from infections and pathogens.
- High in **protein**, supporting tissue development and growth.
- It is low in **fat** and **sugar**, making it easy for a newborn's digestive system to process.
- Acts as a natural **laxative**, helping the baby pass meconium (the first stool) and reducing the risk of jaundice.

Transitional Milk: The Bridge Between Colostrum and Mature Milk

Around the third to fifth day postpartum, the mother's body begins to produce **transitional milk**. This milk serves as a bridge between nutrient-dense colostrum and mature breast milk, adapting to meet the baby's changing needs during the early weeks of life. Transitional milk is higher in fat and calories compared to colostrum, supporting the baby's rapid growth and increased energy demands.

Nutritional Properties:

- It contains more **calories** and increases fat and lactose to support energy needs.

- Rich in **vitamins** like A, E, and C, essential for development and immunity.
- Continues to provide **antibodies** and white blood cells for immune support.

Why It's Important: Transitional milk helps the baby's digestive system adapt to processing larger milk volumes while maintaining robust immune protection.

Mature Milk: Sustained Nutrition

Mature milk typically begins to replace transitional milk around two weeks postpartum and remains the primary source of nutrition for the baby as long as breastfeeding continues. This milk is perfectly balanced to meet the ongoing developmental and energy needs of an infant, adapting in composition over time to support growth and health. It is unique in that it comes in two phases during each feeding:

1. **Foremilk**: Watery and thirst-quenching.
2. **Hindmilk**: Richer and creamier, packed with fat and calories.

Nutritional Properties:

- Contains an optimal balance of **fat, carbohydrates, and protein** to support steady growth and development.
- Rich in **water**, keeping the baby hydrated.
- Provides essential **omega-3 fatty acids** for brain and vision development.
- Continues to deliver **antibodies** and enzymes to boost the baby's immune system.

Why It's Important: Mature milk sustains the baby through critical growth stages, providing the essential nutrients and immune protection needed for long-term health and development. It is uniquely tailored to the baby, constantly adjusting to meet specific needs during the breastfeeding relationship.

Breast Milk adapts uniquely to a baby's needs. When a baby is sick, it increases immune cells and antibodies to fight illness. During growth spurts, milk supply adjusts to meet higher feeding demands. As the baby grows, the milk evolves to provide age-appropriate nutrition. For preterm babies, breast milk contains higher protein levels for growth and enhanced immune-boosting components for added protection.

4.2 MASTERING BREASTFEEDING BASICS: LATCHING AND POSITIONING

Did I mention I'm a certified lactation educator? I love supporting new mamas during their breastfeeding journey. So, when it was my turn to breastfeed my baby, I was pumped with knowledge and confidence. My little Nikola was just like the National Geographic babies I saw in videos, crawling his way to latch onto my breast. But once he latched, it felt like a serpent had bitten me. I screamed, "What the heck was that?"

Since I spoke about how he was misdiagnosed with a cleft palate in the earlier chapter, maybe after several evaluations, I was reinforced —that's a perfectly healthy baby with an intense latch.

It was rough for me. The painful latching lasted for months, and I wanted to quit every single day. On top of that, I wasn't producing as much milk as I had hoped. I have a history of breast surgery, and my milk supply never surpassed 4 ounces during a pumping session. I attended lactation visits where I was told I had hypersensitivity, and it might not go away. But then, one day, when Nikola was 5 months old, the pain just magically disappeared.

I had to accept that my breastfeeding journey would be a dual-feeding experience—both breast and formula. I ended up breast-feeding for 17 months, and that's something I'm very proud of.

Although I've helped so many women exclusively breastfeed their babies, I had to quickly come to terms with the fact that this wouldn't be the case for me. And that's okay. No one is telling you to be perfect at breast-feeding. Contrary to what people who have never had children might think, breastfeeding is not an innate skill that we are born with. It is a learned behavior for both mother and baby. And there are techniques that can help make the learning process easier and more enjoyable.

The Latch

The latch plays a crucial role in breastfeeding. A good latch ensures your baby gets enough milk while keeping you comfortable during feeding. But what does a proper latch look like? Imagine your baby's mouth wide open, covering the nipple and a significant part of the areola, almost like a flower surrounding it. The lips should be flared outward, similar to a fish. I often guide new parents by showing them how to gently adjust the baby's chin and check if the lips are properly flipped outward. It's a small adjustment that often leads to the response, "Wow, that feels so much better!" You should hear a soft sucking sound—clicking or smacking noises could signal a poor latch. If your baby's cheeks dimple or you notice these sounds, it might mean the latch needs some tweaking. Don't worry; this is a normal part of the learning process. You can gently break the suction with your finger, reposition, and try again.

The Positions

Next, let's talk about positions that can make a difference in comfort and effectiveness. The **cradle hold** is a classic choice, where your baby lies across your lap, supported by your arm. The **cross-cradle hold** might be your best bet if you're looking for more control. This involves using the opposite arm to help your baby, allowing your other hand to guide your breast. The **football hold**, where your baby is tucked under your arm like a football, is excellent for those recovering from a C-section or with larger breasts.

For those middle-of-the-night feeds, the **side-lying** position is a lifesaver. This is my favorite position, and I love teaching this to new, exhausted moms who are often tensely holding the baby and could use a much-needed break that echoes a gentle 'We got this". You and your baby lie on your sides facing each other, allowing you to rest as your baby nurses.

Sometimes, no matter how hard you try, latch issues can still pop up. Even one shallow latch can cause nipple soreness, bruising, or pain —it's super common, especially in those early days when you and your baby are figuring things out. A lanolin-based cream or even a little breast milk can work wonders to ease the discomfort. Personally, I swear by those soothing nipple gel pads you can pop in the fridge—they were a lifesaver for me during my breastfeeding journey. Some other things you can try include:

- Ensure your baby's mouth is wide open before latching, like taking a big bite of a sandwich.
- Use breast compression techniques to make latching easier.
- Try different breastfeeding positions to improve latching and find what works best.

If latching continues to be tricky, it might be due to something like a tongue-tie or lip-tie, where the tissue under your baby's tongue or lip limits movement. A lactation consultant or pediatrician can help assess this and guide you through the next steps. You can also find support in your community through resources like La Leche League or explore trusted online sources such as kellymom.com for additional guidance. This is all part of the learning process, and sometimes you will hear the same thing over and over, and then maybe someone else says it a certain way, and it just clicks.

4.3 OVERCOMING BREASTFEEDING CHALLENGES: CLUSTER FEEDING AND SUPPLY ISSUES

Breastfeeding can be a beautiful journey, but it's not always smooth sailing. For some moms, challenges like low milk supply can pop up unexpectedly. This can happen for a variety of reasons—hormonal imbalances, postpartum recovery, or even prior surgeries. But here's an important reminder: struggling with supply has nothing to do with your worth or effort as a mom. Many parents find success with a balanced approach, combining breastfeeding with formula to ensure their baby gets the nutrition they need. This dual feeding method not only helps relieve the pressure of exclusive breastfeeding but also offers flexibility when those unpredictable newborn days hit hard.

What's the Deal with Cluster Feeding?

If you've ever felt like your baby wants to nurse non-stop, welcome to the world of cluster feeding! One moment, they're peacefully snoozing, and the next, they're demanding to nurse every 30 minutes. This behavior is totally normal and often happens during the first few weeks or during growth spurts. It's most common in the late afternoon or evening and can leave you feeling glued to the couch. But don't worry—cluster feeding doesn't mean your milk supply is low. Babies have tiny tummies and are growing fast, so those frequent feedings help meet their nutritional needs and provide comfort as they adjust to the big, wide world.

Creating a Cozy Feeding Space

When you're spending so much time nursing, having a comfy setup can make all the difference. Choose a spot where you can settle in with plenty of pillows for support. Keep snacks, water, and maybe a good book or your favorite show within reach. Staying hydrated and well-fed not only keeps your energy up but also helps with milk production. You might even turn these sessions into a little ritual by adding a favorite playlist or snack—something that makes this time feel special rather than exhausting. And remember, this stage doesn't last forever.

Worried About Milk Supply?

If your baby isn't gaining weight or you're preparing to go back to work, concerns about milk supply are completely normal. Stress, skipping feedings, or hormonal changes can all impact your production. The good news? You can often increase supply by nursing or pumping more frequently—it's all about supply and demand. Some moms also find lactation-friendly foods like oats, fenugreek, or blessed thistle helpful for an extra boost. These strategies might be worth exploring to support your breastfeeding journey.

Nutrition Tips for Nursing Moms

Eating a balanced, nutrient-rich diet is essential while breastfeeding, as your body requires extra calories and nutrients to produce milk. Include a mix of nutrient-rich foods like lean proteins, whole grains, fruits, vegetables, and beneficial fats in your diet. Omega-3 fatty acids, found in foods like salmon, flaxseeds, and walnuts, are particularly beneficial for your baby's brain development. Staying hydrated is equally important—aim to drink water regularly throughout the day, especially during and after nursing sessions.

- **Balanced Diet:** Breastfeeding requires 340-400 extra calories daily. Focus on nutrient-rich foods like dairy, leafy greens (calcium), legumes (iron), and fish/flaxseeds (omega-3s).
- **Quick Snacks:** Try apple slices with almond butter, Greek yogurt with berries, or nuts and dried fruits for easy nutrition.
- **Simple Meals:** Prep dishes like vegetable quinoa salad, chia pudding or stir-fry with brown rice. Batch cook on weekends to save time.
- **Stay Hydrated:** Drink 8-10 cups of fluids daily. Options include water, sparkling water with lime/mint, herbal teas, coconut water, soups, or broths.

- **Lactation Boosters:** Make lactation smoothies (spinach, banana, almond butter, flaxseeds) or energy bites (oats, honey, chia seeds). Include omega-3-rich foods like chia seeds and walnuts.

If you're still worried—maybe your baby isn't gaining weight or has fewer wet diapers—it's a good idea to reach out to a lactation consultant. These experts can provide personalized advice and help with things like pumping techniques or latch issues.

4.4 THE ROLE OF A POSTPARTUM DOULA IN BREASTFEEDING SUCCESS

It's true. You don't have to do this alone. Imagine having someone by your side during the postpartum period who truly understands what you're going through. A postpartum doula provides support that extends beyond physical recovery, offering emotional and practical help, especially with breastfeeding. They listen, reassure, and remind you that you're not alone. From late-night feedings to those first overwhelming days at home, their guidance can make all the difference.

Doulas also provide hands-on breastfeeding support, helping you and your baby find a rhythm. They offer personalized lactation consultations, teaching techniques like proper positioning and latch. Beyond the basics, they help you navigate unexpected challenges, easing the transition into motherhood and boosting breastfeeding success.

Take Penelope, a first-time mom overwhelmed by breastfeeding. With her doula's guidance, she learned techniques to improve her baby's latch, reducing discomfort and building confidence. Her stressful experience turned into an empowering one. Stories like Penelope's show the profound impact doulas can have—offering encouragement and helping new moms overcome challenges.

Finding the right doula is a personal journey. Ask about their training, experience, and breastfeeding support approach. Discuss their availability and how they handle unexpected situations.

Understanding their philosophy will help ensure they're the right fit, giving you a knowledgeable ally.

As we bring this chapter to a close, remember that breastfeeding is about finding what works best for you and your baby. Whether you choose to exclusively breastfeed, supplement with formula or pump milk, having knowledge of the power of womanhood and knowing what your body creates is pretty mind-blowing. The magic of a drop of a colostrum is enough to make me giggle at how powerful we are as women; we create life, and our own bodies make the most perfect substance for a tiny human.

When a mother tells me, "I only breastfed my last baby for a month." I look at them and honor them and say something like, " Well, thank you for breastfeeding for 30 days; you provided that baby with so much gut, and brain set-up in life; you did that, mama. I celebrate mamas breastfeeding their babies on their first day of life. These first drops of colostrum coat their baby's digestive tract.

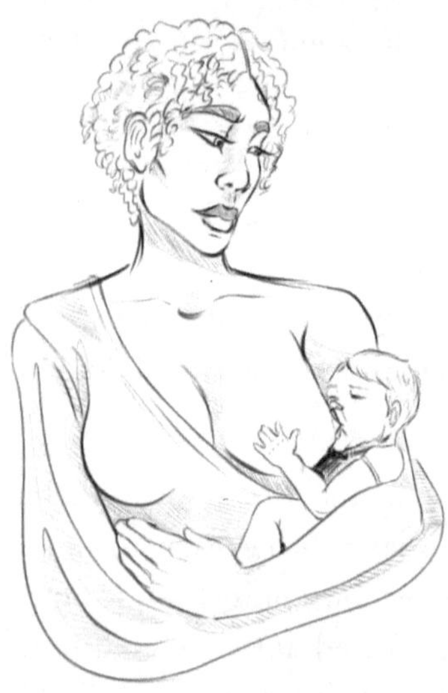

EXERCISE FOR BUILDING YOUR BREASTFEEDING PLAN

Take some time to reflect on your breastfeeding goals, preferences, and feeding choices. Use the prompts and interactive checklist below to create a personalized breastfeeding plan. This exercise is designed to help you feel more prepared and confident about your feeding journey.

Come back to this list and start from the beginning at any point in your journey. This isn't set in stone; you have permission to shift and alter your plan at any time.

1. **Set Your Goals**

   - What are your primary goals for breastfeeding? (e.g., exclusive breastfeeding, combination feeding, pumping, etc.)

   ____

   - How long do you plan to breastfeed? (e.g., 3 months, 6 months, beyond a year?)

   ____

2. **Feeding Choices Checklist**

Create a checklist of your feeding preferences and needs:

   - Do you have specific dietary restrictions to consider while breastfeeding?

   ____

- What are your preferences for formula types or brands, if combination feeding or formula feeding is part of your plan?

- Have you researched different formula options in case breastfeeding is not possible or there is a formula shortage?

Not all formulas are created equal, so it's helpful to stay informed. Take time to research formulas in advance rather than relying on whatever is available at the supermarket or provided at the hospital. Being prepared with options can reduce anxiety and ensure you feel confident about feeding your baby. Use this checklist as a guide when discussing choices with healthcare providers or your support network, aligning your plan with your family's unique needs.

3. **Identify Your Support System**

- Who will be part of your support team? (e.g., partner, family, friends, doula, lactation consultant)

- How will they help you reach your goals? (e.g., preparing meals, providing emotional support, assisting with night feedings)

---

4. Anticipate Challenges

- What potential challenges do you expect to face? (e.g., latching issues, returning to work, low supply)

- What resources or practices could help you overcome these challenges? (e.g., breastfeeding groups, lactation consultations, pumping schedules)

---

5. Communicate Your Plan

- How will you share your plan with your partner, family, or support network?

- What boundaries or requests will you communicate to ensure your plan is respected?

Once you've completed this exercise, review your responses and adapt your plan as needed. Flexibility is key—your needs and circumstances may change, and that's okay.

In this chapter, as we explore breastfeeding and nutrition, remember that your journey is unique and yours to shape. Whether you choose to feed through breast, bottle, or both, the love and intention you bring to nurturing your baby is what truly matters.

My baby, Nikola, in his blue-sky pouch—an Artipoppe baby carrier I had dreamed of for years. It was on my vision board, inspired by a stunning mama in a boho dress carrying her baby in one. My best friend, Preeti, had always promised that when I had a baby, she would gift me that carrier. True to her word, she did. Starting from day six of Nikola's life, I carried him in it for 22 months. He was always close to me, traveling the world chest to chest. I treasure every photo of us together in that carrier.

Each year, approximately 140 million babies are born globally, with 3.6 million of those births occurring in the United States alone. Yet, a majority of new parents feel underprepared; studies show that up to 60% of first-time mothers experience feelings of uncertainty and stress regarding newborn care. From understanding infant sleep patterns to navigating breastfeeding challenges, it's easy to feel overwhelmed without the right guidance.

This chapter will provide practical strategies for caring for your newborn in those early months. We'll explore topics like establishing a feeding routine, managing sleep schedules, and the importance of bonding during developmental milestones. Whether you're a first-time parent or looking for a refresher, the tips shared here are aimed at easing your transition into parenthood and building confidence for the road ahead.

5.1 THE SLEEPING SCHEDULE

We all know the scene: exhausted parents, barely keeping their eyes open, trying to figure out this whole early parenthood thing. I remember meeting Anna, a mom gently rocking her baby to sleep while quietly mumbling a bedtime story, even though she looked ready to pass out herself. Meanwhile, the dad was wrestling with putting together a mobile, staring at the instructions like they were written in code. "We're doing everything we can," Anna said with a tired but determined smile.

As any new parent will tell you, creating a solid sleep routine for a newborn is no easy feat. Those precious moments of quiet can feel like conquering a mountain — but the effort is worth it. Sleep routines aren't just about catching Zs (though, let's be honest, every parent dreams of that sweet, uninterrupted sleep). They're about creating structure in the chaos and helping your baby feel safe and secure.

How to Build a Sleep Routine for Better Rest

A predictable bedtime routine can work wonders for helping your little one wind down. Simple rituals like dimming the lights, singing a soothing lullaby, or giving a warm bath can signal to your baby that it's time to relax. These cues transform bedtime into a cozy nightly show, and your baby is the star performer drifting off into dreamland.

Every baby is unique, and every family has different needs. Some parents prefer gentle approaches, like the "camping out" method, where you gradually reduce your presence in the room as your baby learns to self-soothe. Others may opt for more structured methods, such as the "Ferber" approach, which involves letting your baby cry for short, gradually increasing intervals before offering comfort. The key is to find a method that feels right for your family and your baby's temperament. Experts generally recommend starting sleep training when your baby is around four to six months old, but trust your instincts—no one knows your baby better than you do.

The Curveball That Is Sleep Regression

Just when you think you've nailed the sleep game, along comes sleep regression to throw you off balance. One moment, your baby is sleeping soundly, and you're finally starting to feel like a functioning human again. The next, it's as if you're back to square one with night waking's and endless rocking sessions. Sound familiar?

Sleep regressions are a normal part of development and often occur around three to four months, six months, or eight to ten months. They can even make a cameo appearance in toddlerhood. These disruptions are usually tied to growth spurts or big milestones, like learning to roll over or crawl. While it's frustrating (and exhausting), remember: sleep regressions are temporary phases that typically last two to four weeks.

To weather the storm, stick to your bedtime routine—it provides reassurance for your baby even during chaotic sleep patterns. Patience and persistence are your best friends during these tough nights. Many parents find that white noise or soothing music can help.

Safe Sleep Practices

Safe sleep practices are essential when discussing baby sleep. Placing your baby on their back for sleep has significantly helped lower the risk of Sudden Infant Death Syndrome (SIDS). Make sure the crib is clear of loose blankets, pillows, or soft toys to reduce the chance of suffocation.

Swaddling can be incredibly helpful for calming newborns, as it provides a comforting, womb-like feeling. But once your baby starts showing signs of rolling over, it's time to transition to a sleep sack.

Sleep sacks provide that same cozy warmth without restricting movement, ensuring your baby can sleep safely.

This Too Shall Pass

Parenting is full of highs and lows, and sleep challenges often feel like some of the toughest battles. Whether you're navigating sleep training, managing regressions, or adapting to your baby's changing needs, remember that these phases are temporary. With consistency, patience, and a little trial and error, you'll help your baby develop healthy sleep habits—and maybe even sneak in a well-deserved nap for yourself.

Consider creating a bedtime ritual checklist to ensure consistency. Include steps like "dim lights," "play lullaby," and "read story." This checklist can gently remind you of the soothing sequence that helps signal bedtime, providing a reliable framework for you and your baby.

- Create a calm and dimly lit environment.
- Establish a consistent bedtime.
- Definitely read 1-3 short books
- Sing a lullaby.
- Offer a final feeding if needed to ensure your baby is full.
- Provide a comfort item, like a small blanket or soft toy (only if age-appropriate).
- Practice gentle rocking or cuddling before placing your baby in the crib.
- Lay your baby down while drowsy but awake to promote self-soothing habits.
- Say goodnight with a simple, reassuring phrase.

As you navigate these sleep challenges, know that you're laying the foundation for healthy sleep for your child. Embrace the journey with humor and patience, knowing that restful nights are within reach.

5.2 CRACKING THE CODE TO CLUSTER FEEDING

Picture this: it's 3 a.m., and your baby is wide awake, their tiny tummy grumbling as if they've just finished a marathon. As a new parent, moments like these can feel overwhelming, but establishing a feeding schedule can make all the difference. A good feeding schedule isn't about rigidly watching the clock—it's about understanding your baby's natural rhythms and recognizing their hunger cues.

Understanding Hunger Cues

Newborns communicate their needs in subtle ways. Before the crying starts, look for signs like rooting, lip-smacking, or little fists moving toward their mouth. These cues indicate it's time to feed, and responding promptly helps your baby feel secure and nourished. Watching for these signals allows you to create a responsive feeding routine rather than relying solely on the clock. Balancing feeding times with naps and nighttime sleep isn't always easy—it's an art that requires patience and flexibility.

So, what is cluster feeding?

If you've ever felt like a human buffet, you've likely experienced cluster feeding. This is when your baby nurses more frequently, often in the evenings. While exhausting, cluster feeding serves an essential purpose.

During growth spurts—typically at two to three weeks, six weeks, and three months—your baby's appetite increases to support their rapid growth. These intense feeding periods signal your body to produce more milk, ensuring your baby gets all the nutrients they need. Understanding the "why" behind cluster feeding can help you navigate these moments with more patience and less frustration.

Managing Cluster Feeding

Cluster feeding can be demanding, but there are ways to make it more manageable. Here are some tips to help you through:

1. Prioritize Rest

It can be tempting to catch up on chores, but remember that your well-being is just as important as your baby's. So, take a break.

2. Stay Hydrated and Nourished

Feeding requires energy, so keep water and healthy snacks close during nursing sessions. Staying fueled will help you keep up with your baby's needs.

3. Find Comfortable Feeding Positions

Experiment with positions like cradle, side-lying, or the football hold to find what works best for you and your baby. Comfort can vary day-to-day, so don't hesitate to adjust as needed.

A feeding schedule should be a guide, not a rulebook. Flexibility is key, especially as your baby's needs evolve. What worked during the newborn stage might not suit a three-month-old. Embrace these changes and adapt your routine accordingly.

Baby-led feeding, where you allow your baby to dictate feeding times based on their hunger cues, fosters a positive feeding environment. This approach encourages your baby to eat when hungry and stop when satisfied, promoting healthy growth and development.

By staying attuned to your baby's cues and maintaining a flexible approach, you're setting the foundation for a healthy relationship with food. Feeding times are more than just nourishment—they're moments of connection and care that strengthen the bond between you and your baby.

5.3 BONDING THROUGH SKIN-TO-SKIN AND TUMMY TIME

That first skin-to-skin contact with your baby, the overwhelming love that fills your heart – all of it feels unreal. It is a simple yet powerful way to bond with your newborn in those early days. It helps create a deep connection. When your baby rests against your skin, the warmth and rhythm of your heartbeat provide comfort and security, strengthening your bond in ways words can't describe. This closeness also supports your baby's emotional and physical health by helping regulate their temperature, breathing, and heart rate. It also encourages breastfeeding and boosts milk production, creating a nurturing experience for both of you.

Now, tummy time helps strengthen the muscles in their neck, shoulders, and upper body—muscles they'll need for rolling over, sitting up, and crawling. Tummy time also helps prevent flat spots on the back of your baby's head, which can occur if they spend too much time lying on their back. Start with short sessions, just a minute or two, and gradually increase the time as your baby gets stronger. Aim for several short sessions a day, working up to about an hour total by the time they're three months old.

To make tummy time more enjoyable, try turning it into a fun, engaging activity. Lay your baby on a soft mat and position yourself at their eye level. Use colorful toys or mirrors to capture their attention and encourage them to lift their head. Babies love looking at their own reflections, so mirrors can make tummy time feel like play. Incorporating it into your daily routine as a playful activity can help your baby look forward to it.

Your involvement is key to making these bonding activities meaningful. Talk, sing, or make silly faces to keep your baby entertained during tummy time. If you have older children, involve them too—siblings can show toys to the baby or simply lie nearby, creating a special family moment. These activities are not just about physical development—they're also a chance to build stronger emotional connections with your baby and within your family.

To make it easier for you, I have included an exercise at the end of this chapter to create a tummy time progress chart. This chart will help you track your baby's progress and see how they are improving over time. It can also serve as a fun way to celebrate milestones and achievements.

5.4 RECOGNIZING CUES AND SIGNALS FOR COMMUNICATION

From the very first cry, your baby begins speaking a language all their own—a beautiful symphony of cues and signals designed to tell you exactly what they need. Learning to understand these non-verbal cues is like unlocking a secret code full of tiny gestures, facial expressions, and unique cries. A sharp, piercing wail? Likely hunger. A soft, whimpering cry? Probably tiredness. The key is tuning in. A hungry baby might root around or suck on their fists, while a tired one might rub their eyes or yawn. Discomfort? Look for squirming or arching their back.

When your baby cries, remember—it's not just noise; it's their way of talking to you. Perhaps they're sharing something they're feeling or wanting, or simply releasing the overwhelming flood of daily information and input from their little minds.

Your calm presence and gentle touch can work wonders to soothe them. Try different soothing techniques: swaddle them snugly, rock them gently, or hold them close so they can feel your warmth. Soft shushing sounds or a soothing lullaby might also do the trick. Every baby is unique, so finding what works best may take a little trial and error. The most important thing? Be patient. Every response builds trust and deepens the bond between you and your baby.

Paying attention to your baby's signals not only soothes them in the moment but also supports their emotional development. By consistently addressing their needs, you help them feel secure, loved, and cared for. This process fosters a strong attachment, which plays a key role in forming healthy relationships as they grow. At the same time, teaching your baby to self-soothe is equally essential. Allowing them a moment to fuss without immediate intervention helps them learn to manage their emotions. This doesn't mean ignoring them—it means giving them space to see if they can settle on their own. With time, this approach fosters confidence and emotional resilience.

And don't forget—communication starts long before their first word. Every coo, babble, and giggle are part of their learning journey. When they lock eyes with you, smile, or let out a happy squeal, engage with them! Turn those little sounds into a back-and-forth "conversation." Mimic their coos, exaggerate your facial expressions, and use gestures—they'll love it, and it helps them learn the rhythm of communication. Your playful responses not only entertain but also teach them the fundamentals of human interaction. You're laying the groundwork for their future communication skills while creating priceless moments of connection.

Respond. Engage. Love. The journey of understanding your baby is full of discovery and joy, and every step you take strengthens the bond you share.

5.5 COMMUNICATING WITH YOUR BABY FROM THE WOMB AND BEYOND

Oh, how brilliant tiny humans are. They grow at an exponential rate in the womb. They begin to hear at around 18 weeks. They are already experiencing the world while growing in Mama's belly. The brain is developing at an astonishing rate of over 1 million neural connections per second. They take what they hear and experience as absolute truth.

The benefits of talking, singing, and reading to your baby during pregnancy are instrumental in cultivating healthy brain development. Believe me when I say those little humans are way more intelligent than we give them credit for. Talking to your baby in the womb creates a special bond in which you acknowledge them as whole human beings.

Be intentional about what you consume and who you spend time with during your pregnancy. Babies are always listening, absorbing, and feeling—even in the womb. This isn't to say you can't experience anger or difficult days; it's natural. Rather, it's a reminder to be mindful of the energy and emotions you carry daily. Speak to yourself and your baby with love and positivity.

For example: "Today is a beautiful day. I see gorgeous flowers, the crisp air feels refreshing, and I'm so excited for the day when you'll see it all, too. But until then, I'll tell you all about it."

The world constantly bombards us with information and overstimulation, leaving us almost numb to its effects. By focusing on affirmations, mindfulness, and a sense of safety, you can nurture both your body and your baby. These simple acts help create neural connections that can empower them for a lifetime. Early moments of intentional bonding foster not only security but also a deep connection with your child.

Speak words of encouragement and love:

"Take your time growing, little one. I'm preparing our home for your arrival."

"I know you can feel how deeply loved you are, sweet baby."

"You are so cherished, and so loved."

Even on challenging days, open up to your baby:

"Today, mommy is having a hard day, and that's okay. It's normal to have tough moments. But one thing I know for sure is how much I love you, and that never changes. Let's take deep, calming breaths together. I'll ground myself to ease us both."

Importance of Communication Beyond the Womb

I always tell families in the postpartum unit to talk to their babies about everything they're doing. For example, say, "I'm changing your diaper. The wipe might feel cold—can you feel it?" I encourage parents to introduce their baby to new rooms and explain what's happening throughout the day. Here's an example of how I speak to newborns at the hospital:

"This is Nurse Johaira, and I'm giving you a check-up. First, I'm going to check the temperature under your arm. I know, it's not comfortable—no baby likes a cold thermometer! Okay, your temperature is 98.1, and we're done with that. Now, I need to give you a shot in your thigh. It will hurt, but your mommy and I are here to comfort you."

Some might think this is over the top, but it's not. Talking to your baby builds a foundation of respect and communication. Babies have been developing comprehension and language skills since they were in the womb. While they might seem like blank slates at birth, they've already been learning from you, recognizing your voice and responding to it. Talking to your baby about daily activities—like diaper changes and nap time—engages their brain and helps their cognitive development. Babies are much more perceptive than we often realize, thriving on interaction and connection even in their earliest days.

Encouraging family members to join in this process can create an even richer environment for your baby. Siblings, grandparents, and other loved ones can talk to the baby, helping expand their exposure to language and relationships. Everyday moments, like family dinners, are great opportunities to engage. Narrating what's happening or passing the baby around for cuddles and gentle conversations helps build their understanding of the world and supports brain development.

From birth, babies have an incredible ability to absorb information, showcasing how intelligent and aware they truly are. Treating them with this understanding—through meaningful interactions—nurtures both their cognitive and emotional development. Babies pick up on tone, emotion, and speech patterns, absorbing far more than we often give them credit for. When you talk to your baby, you're not just chatting—you're building a lifelong bond and laying the foundation for their communication skills.

You'll also start noticing what makes your baby feel overstimulated. Every baby is different. Some might feel sensitive to touch, while others crave it. Skin-to-skin bonding is often all they need to feel safe and loved. Babies are comforted by the sounds of the womb—your heartbeat, digestion, and voice vibrations create a reassuring rhythm. After birth, some babies may find a crib too quiet and unfamiliar. They don't need extra stimulation like music or TV; they just need your presence to feel secure and loved.

Touch is essential for babies. Gently caress their hair, back, or feet and observe how they respond. You can't spoil a newborn with too much physical connection—they thrive on it. If you're comfortable, invite family members to share in skin-to-skin bonding. It's a beautiful way to deepen their connection with the baby.

Newborns have blurry vision and can only see about as far as the distance from your breast to your face. This is nature's way of helping them bond with you during feedings. Look at your baby, smile, and speak to them in a calm, loving tone.

I remember doing skin-to-skin with my baby during a Los Angeles heat wave. It was early September, and both of us were sweating. My postpartum body was swollen, and I was shedding extra fluid. Despite the heat, my baby was so happy and peaceful resting on me. We had a small fan to stay cool, and even though it was a lot, it was such a special way to connect. That day, like a superhero, my dear friend stopped by to check in with my favorite salad in hand. She saw us sitting on the chair, pouring sweat, and just took over like a fairy godmother. She made me ice towels and rotated them every 10 minutes with a fresh, cold one. She placed cool towels on my feet. It was one of those moments that stayed with me. Your village can come from anywhere, and my bond with Anne got deeper that day.

Remember, your baby is adjusting to a whole new world outside of the womb. They may feel overwhelmed at times, and that's completely normal. Your presence, touch, and voice can help them feel more secure as they navigate this new environment. As they grow and develop, their needs will also change. It's important to continuously observe and adapt to their individual preferences for touch and stimulation. And the best way to do that is by building a routine.

5.6 THE COMFORT OF ROUTINE COMMUNICATION

Incorporating communication into daily routines is a powerful way to bond with your baby and boost their language and cognitive development. Simple, consistent interactions during activities like feeding, bathing, and bedtime can nurture a sense of security and comfort while supporting learning in meaningful ways.

Using Storytelling and Singing

Reading and singing to your baby from an early age provides countless benefits. Stories and songs not only entertain but also teach, soothe, and strengthen your connection. Something as simple as a lullaby or a short bedtime story can work wonders in fostering comprehension and vocabulary.

Communication with your little humans does not have to be tedious or feel like you're drilling information into them. Speak to them as fully functioning, higher-thinking humans, and you will raise humans who speak to you with the same conviction.

A Bedtime Routine That Teaches and Bonds

Let me share a bedtime ritual we followed every single night—a routine that became a beautiful mix of learning, connection, and comfort for our little one.

We would start with a cheerful greeting every morning:

"Good morning, Nikola. It's a beautiful day. How did you sleep? I'm so happy to see you!"

Come nap time or bedtime, the tone would shift to something soothing yet engaging:

"Okay, little love, it's time for a yummy nap. I love you. Get some good rest."

At bedtime, we'd set out to say goodnight to the house, turning it into a playful and educational moment:

"Okay, Nikola, let's say goodnight to the moon and stars. Is that an airplane I see? Goodnight, moon, stars, and airplane. Goodnight, living room. Goodnight, bike. Goodnight, fridge, stove, and food. Goodnight, toys. Goodnight, bathroom. Let's turn off the bathroom light together — let's count to 5. 1, 2, 3, 4, 5. Goodnight, light!"

Every night, we'd walk through the house together, naming items as we said goodnight. Some nights were slow and relaxed, while others were quick and efficient. No matter the pace, we did it consistently, and the results were incredible. Watching Nikola start to recognize the names of items in our home brought so much joy. By 9 months old, he began counting to 5 during our nightly light-switch countdown. Soon after, we extended the count to 10.

As he grew, the routine evolved. My husband would sometimes open the fridge and say, "Let's see what's inside! Let's say goodnight to it too." These small, playful moments became rich opportunities for vocabulary-building, comprehension, and bonding. The whole process took anywhere from 3 to 10 minutes, and it even gave me a mini mental break to prepare for bedtime. Afterward, we'd read 1-3 small books together, and I'd savor every expression on his little face as I turned off the lights, trying to imprint those moments into my memory forever.

A Simple Phrase with a Big Impact

There was one phrase I made a point to repeat every day:

"It's a beautiful day."

Rain or shine, I'd say it with intention:

"It's a beautiful day — it's cloudy outside."

"It's a beautiful day — it's a sunny day."

"It's a beautiful day — I think it's going to rain soon."

The idea was simple: to frame each day in a positive light, no matter the circumstances. It became a mantra for me and, eventually, for Nikola. By 17 months, he started repeating the phrase back to me: *"It's a beautiful day!"* Hearing those words come from him filled my heart in ways I can't describe.

So, I'd ask him, *"What kind of day is it? Is it a hot, sunny day or a cold, cloudy day?"* And just like that, what started as a simple routine evolved into a loving, interactive exchange—one that reinforced positivity, language skills, and our bond.

The Power of Intentional Routines

Small, intentional routines like these can create lasting connections and teach invaluable lessons. Whether it's counting down to turn off the lights, naming objects, or simply repeating positive phrases, these moments are more than just habits—they're opportunities to nurture your baby's growth and cherish the journey of parenthood.

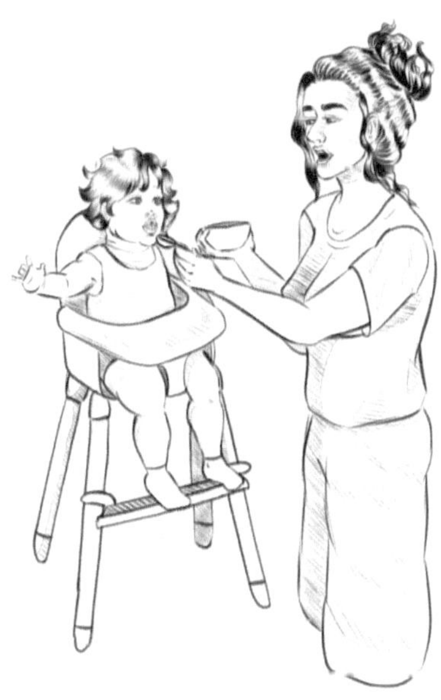

Exercise: Building A Tummy Time Progress Chart

Keep track of your baby's tummy time sessions with an easy-to-use chart! Use it to log how long each session lasts and document exciting milestones, like lifting their head or pushing up on their arms. This simple activity lets you celebrate your baby's progress while building a stronger connection.

How to Start:

1. Grab a notebook or create a chart digitally.
2. Use columns for the date, tummy time duration, and milestones.
3. Update it daily or weekly to see their progress.
4. Create a checklist for important development milestones.
5. Celebrate their achievements and keep track of any concerns or delays.

CHAPTER 6

LOVE, PARTNERSHIPS, AND INTIMACY

While childbirth and postpartum care are often seen as solely a woman's domain, research has shown that having a supportive partner involved can positively impact the physical and emotional health of both mother and baby. Partners who are actively involved in the process have been found to provide crucial support, decrease stress levels for mothers, and promote positive bonding experiences between father and child.

I will be the first to admit that it was really hard to reconnect with my partner since having a baby. I've loved him since I was 21, and we always find our way back to each other. While we share beautiful moments, like looking at each other in awe of our baby, it's been challenging to rebuild the intimate connection we once had. I feel like I'm finally starting to come back to "us." I realize now that I was the one who was emotionally withdrawn, pouring my whole heart into this new chapter of being a parent.

According to a 2020 study published in the Journal of Perinatal Education, fathers who are involved in postpartum care are associated with a 27% reduction in maternal anxiety and an overall improvement in family bonding. I'll never forget a young couple I worked with during a particularly challenging postpartum period. The mother was recovering from an emergency C-section and was unable to perform many tasks in those critical early days. Her partner had previously admitted to being terrified of hospitals, and yet I remember his huge hands swaddling his newborn for the first time. The gentle care and attention he gave to the new presence in his life was evident. He learned to handle diaper changes, practiced skin-to-skin contact, supported the mother with breastfeeding, and actively sought out ways to learn how to care for their baby. He even attended lactation support sessions to assist with feeding. Days later, he told me, "I didn't know I had it in me, but now I'm so proud of what we've done together." His active participation not only strengthened their partnership but also created a nurturing environment for their new baby to thrive. And let me tell you - this dynamic of partner involvement is vital to the well-being of both mother and child.

In this chapter, we will explore the various ways in which partners can be involved and support their partners during the postpartum period. From practical tasks like household chores and baby care, to emotional support and communication, there are many ways for partners to play an active role in this special time. We will also discuss the importance of taking care of the connection. The goal is not only to ease the burden on new mothers but also to create a stronger family unit where both parents are empowered and actively participating in the care of their child. As they say, it takes a village - and having a supportive partner by your side can make all the difference

6.1 THE IMPORTANCE OF PARTNER SUPPORT IN PARENTING

As parents, it's easy to get caught up in daily tasks and responsibilities, but it's important to remember the importance of bonding and active involvement in your baby's life. Today's family configurations vary widely, including single parents, domestic partnerships, and same-sex relationships, each with its distinct strengths and challenges. Often, the person offering support isn't a spouse but a dedicated friend or relative, ready to embrace the joys and challenges of parenthood alongside you.

In many cultures, family goes beyond parents and children. Child-rearing is often a shared effort, with grandparents, aunts, uncles, and neighbors all playing active roles. This communal approach offers valuable support but can also bring challenges as different generations mix their parenting styles. This used to be the norm in Western societies, but as extended families have dispersed and communities have become more fragmented, the role of parenting has often fallen solely on the parents themselves.

Now, partners are taking on more active roles than ever before. Gone are the days when parenting was considered solely a mother's domain. According to recent studies, fathers spend three times as much time with their children as they did in the 1960s. This evolution reflects a growing recognition of the importance of shared parenting responsibilities, not only for the child's well-being but also for the relationship's health. This shift is not just about dividing tasks but about fostering deeper emotional connections with the child from an early age.

The numbers tell an interesting story. According to a Pew Research survey, 57% of dads now feel like they're doing a good job as parents —a big shift from previous decades. This reflects a growing cultural shift toward recognizing and supporting different family roles. But it's not all smooth sailing. As partners take on more at home, they're also juggling challenges like balancing work and family or navigating the emotional ups and downs of parenthood together. And while it's a step in the right direction, there is still much work to be done in terms of breaking traditional gender roles and promoting true equality in parenting responsibilities.

6.2 THE SUPPORT GAP BETWEEN US

Sometimes, your partner might think they're doing everything right, but you still don't feel supported—and it's not just about chores like taking out the trash or doing the dishes. It's about emotional support, especially during the postpartum period. Navigating this time can feel like learning a new dance, where both partners are trying to find their rhythm, but each person is listening to their own genre of music.

It's common to encounter a "support gap" where expectations and reality don't quite match. This often stems from differing assumptions about postpartum recovery. One partner might expect a quick bounce back, while the reality of physical recovery and emotional overwhelm is far more complex. Miscommunication can further widen this gap. One of you might crave quiet time to process, while the other seeks constant connection and interaction—it can feel like you're tuning in to completely different radio stations.

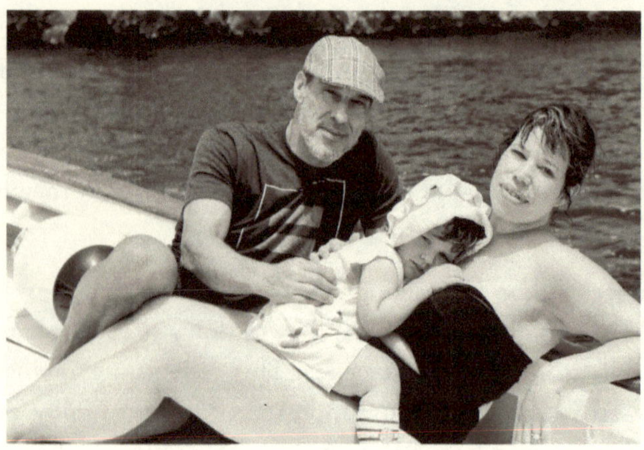

Eric, Nikola, and me — June 21, 2024 Capri, Italy | Photo by a lovely woman who was determined to capture all three of us on the boat with a 50mm lens—your perseverance is so appreciated Take the family trip. Wear the bathing suit. Take up space. Be unapologetically you—your joy deserves to be seen.

Then there's the multitasking challenge. Caring for a newborn often demands juggling multiple tasks at once, but not everyone is naturally wired for it. Some partners are great at focusing on one thing but struggle with switching gears quickly. Multitasking is a skill that can be learned, like riding a bike—with patience, practice, and a little teamwork. By recognizing and addressing these gaps together, you can build stronger support and truly show up for each other during this life-changing chapter.

Do you know what you need to bridge this gap?

It starts with open and honest communication. Share your needs with your partner, both emotional and physical. Open discussions are key to bridging this gap. Imagine sitting down with your partner, coffee in hand, and having an open, honest conversation about your needs and expectations. And you can't just do it once and call it a day; you need to regularly check in. Because the goal is to make these conversations as natural as brushing your teeth—part of your routine. Setting aside time for a weekly discussion, like a standing date amidst the chaos of parenting, can help you both pause, connect, and realign.

Then comes listening with empathy. Truly listening to your partner —actively and without judgment—goes beyond hearing their words; it's about understanding the emotions behind them. Sharing daily experiences isn't just venting; it's a way to intertwine your perspectives. This practice helps foster compassion and strengthens the bond between you, creating an environment where both partners feel valued and supported.

Equitable support is the foundation of a strong partnership. Dividing responsibilities doesn't mean splitting everything 50/50—it's about playing to each partner's strengths. If one of you loves cooking while the other thrives at organizing, lean into those abilities to turn household tasks into a collaborative effort, not a chore. For example, rotating nighttime baby duties ensures both partners get rest and reinforces a sense of teamwork. Think of it as passing the baton in a relay race—working together to avoid burnout.

Ultimately, overcoming support gaps in a relationship means recognizing and valuing each partner's unique contributions. A strong partnership is built on mutual respect, shared responsibilities, and open communication.

Of course, it's one thing to imagine a calm, productive conversation about your needs; it's another to try having that conversation while sleep-deprived, frustrated, or feeling unsupported. And that's okay. Not every conversation will go smoothly, and things can get messy.

So, let's look at some of the ways you can effectively communicate with your partner about your expectations and feelings.

6.3 THE ART OF TALKING & LISTENING

Effective communication is key in navigating new parenthood. Clear, honest dialogues help you and your partner express thoughts, emotions, and expectations, building trust and understanding. Each conversation strengthens your bond, helping you overcome challenges together. Setting and discussing clear goals—whether for your family or individual aspirations—keeps you aligned and focused, even amid life's unpredictability.

How can you do this?

Start by focusing on something positive: "I love how connected you are with our baby—you're such a wonderful parent." Then, express your feelings: "I'm feeling _________, and I think we need to figure out how to bring more balance to this area."

If you start a conversation with, "*You* don't help enough," or, "*You* always make a mess," you're immediately placing blame and creating defensiveness. Instead, try using "I" statements to express how something is affecting you personally: "I feel overwhelmed when the house is messy." This can help your partner understand you without feeling attacked themselves.

Next, listen to their response with an open mind. Even if you don't agree, acknowledging and understanding their emotions can help de-escalate any tension and create a more productive conversation. And remember, communication is a two-way street; be sure to actively listen and respond with empathy as well.

Active listening is about genuinely understanding your partner's perspective, reflecting on what you've listened to, and asking clarifying questions. Doing this validates their feelings and shows you're engaged and invested in resolving any issues.

The postpartum period can bring exhaustion and stress, creating communication challenges that complicate even basic conversations. Sleep deprivation often distorts meaning, turning harmless remarks into perceived criticism or disinterest. To navigate this, cultivate patience and reflect before responding. Avoid assumptions—direct communication is key to clearing up misunderstandings and preventing minor issues from escalating.

Let me keep it real—the first year of parenthood was tough on my relationship. After nearly two decades with my partner, we suddenly felt like two grumpy roommates in survival mode. Without family nearby (we live in California), we were overwhelmed. I was exhausted, frustrated, and felt like I was bearing the entire mental load. My partner was truly wonderful and invaluable, helping so much with the baby and around the house, but it still never felt like enough. I longed for a village and unfairly placed those expectations on one person who was also trying to adjust to this sleep-deprived reality.

Maintaining a healthy relationship during this time requires effort and adaptability. Regular check-ins, even brief ones over coffee or during a walk, help keep you aligned as partners. Use these moments to adjust roles and responsibilities—like alternating bedtime routines or grocery shopping—to ensure the load is shared. Flexibility fosters mutual support and prevents resentment.

Open and honest communication is the foundation of resilience. By working together and staying adaptable, you can navigate the challenges of parenting while strengthening your relationship, creating a partnership that thrives even through life's toughest changes.

6.4 SHARING THE LOAD TOGETHER

My family would joke about how it would be when all the attention was no longer on me. But jokes on them—I never wanted or desired anything as much as creating human life and watching them grow.

During that first year, it was really rough adjusting to the balance of parenting. I feel like once my baby started communicating, playing, and interacting, my husband became more of an equal partner in the parenting game. But during that adjustment period, I was pissed—truly upset that I didn't feel like I had someone equally sharing the parenting responsibilities.

Now that I have a full-on toddler—I've kicked back a lot. And although my husband might feel like he's taking on more of the work than I am, I've realized that's just how parenthood is. We take turns carrying the heavier load, and that's okay.

The important thing is that we communicate and support each other in this journey. We make time for just the two of us, even if it's just a quick date night at home after our child goes to bed. We celebrate each other's small victories and offer words of encouragement when things get tough. And most importantly, we strive to maintain the love and connection that brought us together in the first place.

At one point, I talked to my partner about how unbalanced parental duties felt. He insisted he was already maxed out, even offering to list everything he did. While I never got that list, the conversation sparked a change. Looking back, creating a list together could've helped us divide tasks more fairly.

Teamwork is what turns a household from surviving to thriving. Celebrating small wins—like getting the baby to sleep through the night or enjoying an uninterrupted meal—brings partners closer and fosters collaboration. Supporting each other's parenting styles is just as vital. Respecting differences, whether it's handling tantrums or bedtime routines, strengthens the parenting experience by turning diverse perspectives into assets.

6.5 LOVE NOTE TO THE DADS

There are so many amazing dads in my community who show up in powerful, tender ways. The more I look for it, the more I see—it's truly inspiring.

When you mess up, when patience runs thin, and when the day pulls more from you than you had to give—offering an apology is a quiet kind of bravery.

Saying, *"I'm learning too."* becomes its kind of love language.

And whispering, *"Tomorrow, I'll be a little softer, a little sillier, a little better,"* plants seeds of healing in both of you.

This work you're doing—it echoes. It matters. It grows.

And the exact honest, tender words you offer your child can strengthen your partnership.

Because growth, love, and repair are part of the journey—not just with your baby, but with each other.

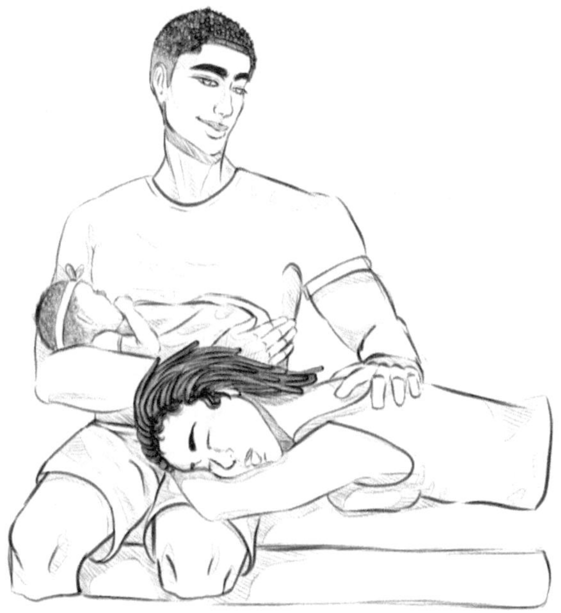

6.6 KEEPING THE SPARK ALIVE

Let's face it - parenthood can be exhausting and the demands of raising young children can take its toll on a romantic relationship. You don't feel your best after being up all night with a crying baby, and date nights become a distant memory. But maintaining a strong connection with your partner is not a luxury but a necessity.

Emotional and physical intimacy are key to maintaining a strong relationship, especially during the challenges of parenthood. Emotional closeness builds family stability and creates a supportive environment for your child, while physical connection strengthens your bond and provides much-needed comfort as you navigate this new chapter together.

One effective way to reconnect is through regular date nights. Whether at home or out, these moments allow you to step away from parenting roles and focus on each other. At-home options can be simple yet meaningful—turn your living room into a cozy space for a movie night or cook a meal together and enjoy the process. If childcare is available, plan outings like a walk in the park, coffee at your favorite spot, or even a short road trip to rekindle the excitement that brought you together.

Postpartum intimacy often comes with challenges. Physical changes, exhaustion, and shifting priorities can affect libido and lead to feelings of disconnection. Open communication with your partner is essential—discuss your needs, boundaries, and emotions to create a supportive space for intimacy to naturally rebuild. Body image concerns are also common, but sharing these feelings can foster empathy and reassure you that your worth goes beyond physical appearance.

Small, thoughtful gestures go a long way in strengthening your bond. Write a quick love note, send a sweet text, or plan a surprise like your partner's favorite meal or a relaxing bath. Expressing appreciation for everyday acts like making coffee or handling chores can also reinforce your connection and show your gratitude. These simple actions build a strong foundation of mutual care and affection.

6.7 LETTING GO OF PRESSURE, HONORING YOUR BODY

It's completely normal if you're not ready for physical intimacy after having a baby. You may feel like you have no desire for it—and that's valid. Your body has been through something monumental; sometimes, it just needs to be left alone. The shift into new motherhood can leave you feeling physically, emotionally, and energetically spent. You don't have to force yourself to do anything you're not ready for. The most important thing is that you feel safe enough to talk openly with your partner. Ask for space if you need it. If it helps, gently explain that it's not about no longer being attracted to them—it's about needing time and room to reconnect with yourself before feeling ready to connect with anyone else. Your needs matter. You deserve that grace.

6.8 FOR PARTNERS: STAYING CLOSE WITHOUT PRESSURE

This time can feel confusing or even a little hurtful for partners, but know this: your person still loves you. They may be completely overwhelmed, touched out, or navigating a deep physical and emotional healing process. Instead of focusing solely on when things will "go back to normal," try shifting the goal to building emotional safety and connection. Little acts of intimacy can go a long way—holding hands during a walk, a warm hug at the end of the day, or a gentle kiss each morning. These moments help build trust, closeness, and reassurance without pressure. Be patient, be present, and remind them through your actions that they are loved just as they are in every phase of this transition. True intimacy starts with feeling seen and supported.

6.9 REDEFINING INTIMACY IN THE POSTPARTUM SEASON

Intimacy after birth doesn't have to mirror what it once was. In fact, *redefining intimacy* during this season of change can become one of the most powerful ways to stay connected while honoring each other's evolving needs.

Maybe intimacy now means taking a quiet shower together without interruptions.

Maybe it's your partner bringing you a snack while you nurse or gently rubbing your shoulders during the baby's nap.

Maybe it's simply laughing together in the middle of a chaotic diaper blowout.

Real intimacy is built in these small, consistent acts of care, tenderness, and attention.

It's not about rushing back to "normal"—it's about creating a *new normal* rooted in patience, respect, and mutual understanding.

There is no perfect timeline for when everything will "return"—and that's okay. Love often deepens most not in the easy moments, but in the messy, uncertain, in-between spaces. If communication ever feels overwhelming or hard to navigate, reaching out to a postpartum counselor or couples' therapist can offer guidance and support. Sometimes, the strongest bridges are built when we allow ourselves to be supported.

Ultimately, prioritizing your relationship after birth isn't just about keeping romance alive—it's about nurturing a stable, loving foundation for your growing family. A strong, connected partnership becomes a sanctuary where your child can feel safe, secure, and thrive.

Before we dive into balancing work and family life, let's take a moment to honor the importance of physical closeness, emotional communication, and the ongoing journey of reconnecting with your partner in a way that meets you both where you are—right here, right now.

EXERCISE: UNDERSTANDING YOUR FAMILY DYNAMICS

1. Vent and Release

Start by journaling freely about any frustrations or challenges you're experiencing. Write about areas where you feel you could use more support. Let your thoughts flow without judgment.

____

____

____

____

____

2. Explore Your Family's Unique Dynamics

Once you've cleared your mind, reflect on your family's unique dynamics. Consider the evolving roles each family member has taken on and the cultural influences that have shaped your parenting approaches. How have these dynamics impacted your family interactions?

____

____

____

3. Harmonize Parenting Styles

Reflect on your partner or support network and think about how your parenting styles complement each other. Consider how these differences or similarities create balance in your child's upbringing. Are there areas where you could align more effectively?

____

____

____

4. Identify Strengths and Growth Areas

Reflect on the strengths within your family relationships and note areas where growth is possible. Consider how these insights can help foster a deeper connection and understanding within your family.

____

____

____

5. Create a Family Mantra

Together, craft a family mantra that reflects your family values. This can serve as a guiding principle for your collective journey. For example:

"In this family, we are open to growing and evolving. We choose kindness, love, and respect in all we do. Together, we believe in our capacity for growth and understanding."

Use this exercise to gain clarity, strengthen bonds, and embrace your family's path with love and adaptability.

____

____

A GENTLE GIFT FOR YOUR JOURNEY

Motherhood transforms everything—and healing deserves support.

To walk with you through this season, I created something special:

The Gentle Postpartum Reset — simple practices for grounding, healing, and reconnecting with yourself after becoming a mother.

Download your free guide here: www.johairamichelle.com/free

For daily inspiration, honest reflections, and community, follow along:

TikTok: @allthingspostpartumbook

If these words have already touched your heart, I would be honored if you left a review to help another mother find her way.

Scan Here to go Directly to
the Review Page

Your voice has the power to light someone else's path.

CHAPTER 7

WORK-LIFE BALANCE AND RETURNING TO WORK

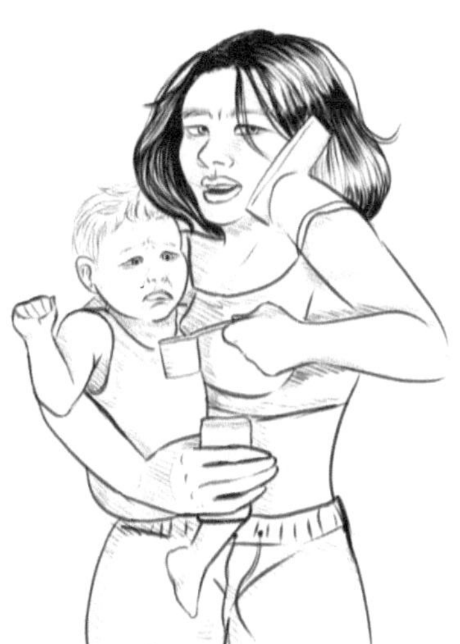

Motherhood is definitely one of the hardest and most time-consuming jobs you will ever do. But you had a whole personality before becoming a mom, before becoming responsible for someone else's life. You might be in the middle of a career you had worked hard for, or you might be a stay-at-home mom. Either way, the decision to work post-baby can be daunting.

The transition from a full-time mom to having two full-time jobs can be overwhelming. And if you're like me, who loves being a mom, loves caring for new babies coming into the world, and is always doing some sort of creative project—whether it's directing a music video or creating a wellness event. Be prepared to feel like you are being pulled from all directions and stretched to your limits.

The days of focusing solely on your baby are suddenly packed with emails, meetings, and commutes. It's a tough transition—shifting from the round-the-clock needs of a newborn to juggling deadlines and responsibilities outside the home. It won't always be easy; there will be moments of tears and frustration, but with some planning, you can navigate this challenging era and find a rhythm that works for both you and your family.

In this chapter, we will discuss the importance of finding a work-life balance as a new mom and strategies for returning to work after having a baby. We will also explore tips for managing guilt, setting boundaries, and prioritizing your well-being while juggling multiple roles. Whether you are a first-time mom or a seasoned pro, this chapter will provide valuable insights on how to navigate the delicate balance between motherhood and career.

7.1 MASTERING MATERNITY LEAVE

I returned to work after my maternity leave ended but felt completely unprepared. Walking the halls where I worked triggered PTSD, and I ultimately had to ask my doctor for extended time off. I definitely wasn't ready, but I was able to get 3 more months off, and that additional time made all the difference in having a more balanced return to work.

Becoming a mom is a life-changing journey, and balancing the demands of motherhood and work is an adjustment. The truth is, there's no perfect formula. The goal isn't perfection; it's finding a balance that works for you and your family. But you can take steps to make the process smoother.

Know Your Rights and Benefits

You need to advocate like a mother! I've heard shocking things, like, "Back in my day, I pumped in a bathroom stall," or my new boss telling me on my first day back, "Well, it's just a reality—sometimes you just won't have time to pump."

In this case, knowledge is power. You need to know that you have legal rights in place to protect you as a new mother. In the U.S., the Family and Medical Leave Act (FMLA) allows eligible employees up to 12 weeks of unpaid leave. However, not everyone qualifies, so it's important to check your eligibility and see how FMLA aligns with your company's specific benefits.

Additionally, familiarize yourself with the Pregnancy Discrimination Act (PDA), which protects against unfair treatment due to pregnancy. Some states even offer additional leave benefits, so a little research can go a long way. If you have short-term disability insurance, this can help supplement your income during your leave. Just keep in mind that you typically need to have this insurance in place at least three months before getting pregnant to qualify.

Financial preparation is another key part of the puzzle. Think about how your income might shift during maternity leave and create a budget to manage expenses. Make a list of anticipated costs like baby gear, healthcare, and everyday items, then map out a plan that works for your family.

The ideal time to gather intel on your rights and what you might need is before you're pregnant. But if that ship has sailed, the second-best time is NOW. The better prepared you are, the less stressful things will be.

Navigating Leave Policies

Let's be honest—figuring out maternity leave paperwork, benefits, and policies can feel like navigating a maze. Outdated systems, long hold times, and confusing instructions can leave you feeling frustrated. Trust me, it's a universal hassle that needs major improvement.

Start by reviewing your company's policies and preparing a list of questions. Don't hesitate to ask for clarification—*multiple times* if needed. Scheduling a meeting with your HR department can provide the answers you need. Use this time to discuss your leave plans, ensure you understand your entitlements, and clear up any uncertainties.

For those who might not know, the EDD (Employment Development Department) is the agency in California responsible for administering unemployment benefits and disability insurance. As a new mother, I thought this resource would help me.

Let me make one thing clear: the EDD phone system is a complete disaster. I would often wait on hold for 40 minutes only to hear an operator say, "We've met the limit for callers today. Goodbye." If you're in the U.S., I highly recommend finding your local EDD office—**somewhere you can speak to an actual person.** Arrive early, expect to stay 4–6 hours, and just get it done. I had to go three times during my postpartum period, but each visit eventually resolved what I needed.

Creating a work transition plan can also make a big difference. Writing everything down clears space in your mind for what matters most. Outline your current projects, upcoming deadlines, and any critical information your colleagues will need while you're away. Share this in a detailed handover document, and identify a reliable point of contact for ongoing tasks.

This thoughtful preparation not only supports your team but also gives you *peace of mind* as you step into maternity leave.

Planning for Your Return

As you prepare for maternity leave, it's a great time to think about what your work life will look like when you return. The workplace is evolving, and flexible arrangements like remote work or part-time schedules are becoming more common. Talk to your employer about options that allow you to balance your job with your new responsibilities at home.

Advocating for your needs is also important—especially if you're breastfeeding. The PUMP for Nursing Mothers Act requires employers to provide break time and a private space (not a bathroom) for expressing milk. This knowledge can save you any awkward conversations down the track. And can empower you to know what you are entitled to in the workplace.

While on leave, be sure to connect with your colleagues and stay updated on any changes in the workplace. This will help you ease back into work smoothly when the time comes. And don't forget to take care of yourself during this transition period. Maternity leave can be physically and emotionally taxing, so make sure you find ways to prioritize self-care and ask for support if needed.

So, no matter what anyone tells you, if you're not ready, advocate for yourself and ask for more time off. In the end, clear communication, thorough preparation, and knowing your rights will empower you to make decisions that suit your family and career. Remember, you're not alone in this journey—lean on your support system and take each step one day at a time.

7.2 TRANSITIONING BACK TO BOSS MODE

Heading back to work after maternity leave can feel like walking a tightrope—equal parts excitement, anxiety, and a sprinkle of guilt. But with a little planning and the right mindset, it doesn't have to feel like a high-stakes circus act. Here's how to navigate this transition with grace, a touch of humor, and, most importantly, your sanity intact.

Jumping back into full-time work right away can feel overwhelming, so consider easing in. Many workplaces are open to a **phased return** —shorter hours or a few days a week. If possible, time your return for a less hectic period at work. For example, avoid coming back from leave during a major project deadline or peak season. This will give you some breathing room to get into the swing of things and avoid feeling bombarded with tasks right away.

The next thing to take care of is your **mom's guilt**. You know what I'm talking about, that nagging feeling in the back of your mind that you're somehow not doing enough for your child or family. That feeling is hard to kick back, especially as a new mother. You might worry about leaving your baby or feel torn between missing them and secretly enjoying your coffee while it's still hot. Here's the truth: it's okay to feel both.

Let go of the idea that you need to be perfect. Focus on what matters most each day, whether it's delivering on that work deadline or making it home in time for bedtime cuddles. Perfection is overrated —your best is more than enough.

And I know people talk about having "work-life balance" when the truth is, they are not opposing forces to balance. Think **integration** instead. Look for ways your professional and personal lives can support each other. Maybe your company hosts family-friendly events, or you can bring a little work productivity into personal time by planning meals during your lunch break.

It's also worth finding creative ways to maximize your time. Use your commute for quick calls or to catch up on tasks (just not while driving, please). These little adjustments can free up time for what really matters—your family, your work, and yes, even a little time for yourself.

The key to transitioning back to work is finding a rhythm that feels natural. It's not about juggling everything perfectly—it's about finding a flow that works for you. Manage your expectations, find moments to laugh at the chaos, and remember that this is just a phase of life —it won't last forever.

Lastly, you don't have to do it all alone. Lean on your support system. Whether it's family, friends, or a trusted childcare provider, having help can make all the difference. Consider asking a family member to help with childcare, or at the very least, someone who can listen when you need to vent.

Other working moms are a goldmine of advice and reassurance. They've been there, done that and probably know first-hand how to balance work and a new baby. Whether it's swapping scheduling hacks or laughing over shared chaos, their insights can be a sanity-saver.

Returning to work after maternity leave can be a big transition, but it doesn't have to drown you. With some planning, support, and a little self-compassion, you'll settle into a routine that works for you—imperfect, but completely your own.

7.3 TIME MANAGEMENT HACKS FOR WORKING MOMS

I know I gave you the blanket advice of "integration" earlier, but let's get a little more specific. Time management is crucial for all of us, but it becomes even more important when you're juggling work and motherhood. Here are some time management hacks that helped me stay organized and productive:

1. Prioritize What Really Matters

The first step to effective time management is learning what truly deserves your attention. Use a daily planner to map out your tasks, but don't just list everything—focus on your top three priorities for the day. These should be the tasks that will have the biggest impact, whether it's a work deadline, an important family activity, or simply carving out time for yourself. This approach ensures you channel your energy into what matters most, rather than trying to do every-thing at once.

2. Embrace Time-Blocking

Time-blocking is a lifesaver for busy moms. Instead of multitasking (which often leads to more stress), allocate specific chunks of time for each activity—work, family, and personal time. For example, set aside 30 minutes in the morning for focused work, an hour in the evening for family dinner, and even 10 minutes for a quick breather. This structure keeps your day on track and prevents you from feeling overwhelmed by competing demands.

3. Cut Down on Distractions

Distractions are one of the biggest time-wasters. Think of all those moments spent scrolling your phone or reacting to notifications. Sarah used to fall into the trap of doom-scrolling before bed, telling herself she'd check Instagram for "just five minutes." An hour later, she was still watching funny videos—and losing precious time, she could have spent sleeping or relaxing. Sound familiar? Combat this habit by turning off unnecessary notifications and setting phone-free zones during critical moments, whether it's during family time or focused work hours. A dedicated, clutter-free workspace—like a simple corner desk—is also a great way to minimize interruptions and stay on task.

4. Streamline Household Chores

Household responsibilities can feel never-ending, but there are ways to make them more manageable. For starters, meal prepping can save countless hours during the week. Spend a couple of hours on the weekend making meals like soups, casseroles, or pasta dishes that can be portioned and reheated. This reduces the stress of figuring out what to cook every day.

Another game-changer? Delegate. Create a family chore schedule and assign age-appropriate tasks to your kids and partner. This not only lightens your load but teaches responsibility and teamwork. Consider using a family calendar app to track chores and coordinate everyone's activities, so nothing slips through the cracks.

5. Make Room for Self-Care

Taking care of yourself isn't selfish—it's essential. It's easy to push self-care to the back burner when life feels overwhelming, but even a small effort can go a long way. A 15-minute walk or quick stretch session can boost your energy and reset your mind. Find small moments to recharge, whether it's sipping tea in silence or reading a chapter of a book. Self-care isn't about luxury; it's about ensuring you have the energy to show up fully for your family, work, and yourself.

6. Use a Weekly Planner

A weekly planner can be your secret weapon. Whether you buy one or create your own, make sure it includes sections for work goals, family time, and self-care. Seeing everything laid out visually helps you manage your time more efficiently and ensures you don't overlook important commitments. Treat this planner as your tactical guide, keeping you organized and intentional about how you use your time.

7.4 DRAWING THE LINE BETWEEN WORK & FAMILY

Imagine wrapping up your workday when your phone buzzes with yet another after-hours email. Your mind is already at home with your family, but the pull to respond feels unavoidable. Work boundaries aren't just about saying no—it's about protecting your well-being.

Start by limiting after-hours communication. Decide when to stop checking emails and stick to it. Communicate these boundaries with your team so they understand and respect your priorities. Discuss workload expectations with your supervisor to ensure they align with your capacity, reducing unnecessary stress and improving your focus outside work.

Many struggle with saying no, especially in environments where being constantly available feels expected. But declining tasks that conflict with family time is essential. Frame it positively: instead of a flat "no," try saying, "I'm focused on finishing my current projects and can't take on more right now." This shows dedication while maintaining your limits.

Prioritizing tasks is equally important. Focus on high-impact or urgent duties. Direct your energy where it matters most—professionally and personally.

Advocating for family-friendly policies is another vital step. Use HR meetings or informal discussions to push for changes like flexible hours, improved parental leave, or on-site childcare. These initiatives can ease the burden of balancing work and family for everyone.

Build a supportive network of colleagues who share similar values. Work together to promote work-life balance and advocate for each other when needed. Organize discussions or workshops where employees can share strategies and experiences. This not only raises awareness but fosters a culture that values and respects family commitments.

By setting boundaries, advocating for better policies, and fostering a supportive workplace, you can create balance and thrive in both work and family life. In the next chapter, we'll explore self-care and mindfulness practices to help you manage the demands of motherhood and maintain your well-being.

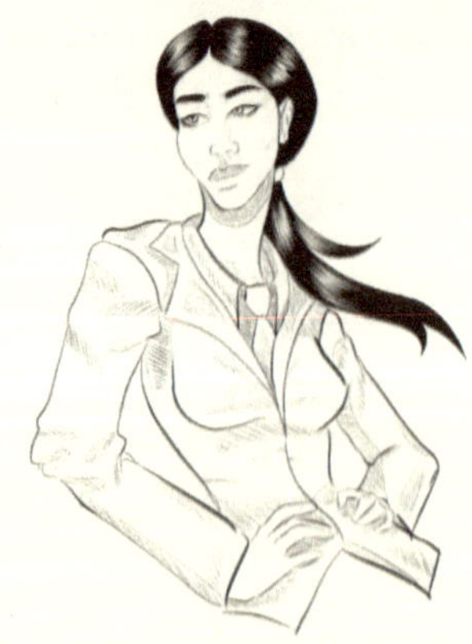

EXERCISE: MATERNITY LEAVE PLANNING CHECKLIST

Goal: Create a personalized maternity leave plan to help you prepare effectively and ensure a smooth transition.

Step 1: Research and Write Down Key Information

- Research your legal rights regarding maternity leave.
- Review your company's maternity leave policies.
- Look into financial assistance options, including Paid Family Leave and EDD.

Step 2: Create a Financial Plan

- Calculate your expected expenses during leave.
- Determine how much financial support you'll need and where it will come from (savings, benefits, etc.).

Step 3: Plan Workplace Communication

- Schedule a meeting with HR to clarify policies and expectations.
- Draft a work transition plan to outline how your responsibilities will be managed during your leave.

Step 4: Develop a Timeline

- Set deadlines for completing the above tasks.
- Include key dates, such as when to notify your employer and when to apply for benefits.

Step 5: Review and Refine the Plan

- Double-check your checklist to make sure nothing is missed.
- Ask clarifying questions.

By completing this exercise, you'll have a clear roadmap to guide you through the maternity leave process, ensuring a smooth and less stressful transition into this exciting new chapter.

CHAPTER 8
SELF-CARE HACKS FOR A CHAOTIC WORLD

When I had my baby, I never truly stopped doing the things I love. At just 2 months old, with my baby in my arms, I held a screening for a music video I wrote, starred in, and directed called "RONA." I also showcased my pandemic music video trilogy, which I had created during the pandemic to promote vaccines. In fact, I was 7 months pregnant with my baby, Nikola, when I created "RONA." I felt so proud of myself that day—newly postpartum, swollen, and embodying a version of myself that was strong and determined. During the Q&A, I spoke with confidence and conviction. That moment, for me, was self-care.

It reminded me that I can still create art. Even though life looks very different now, the seeds I've planted are growing roots. About 3 weeks postpartum, I also made it to a film screening of one of my music videos. It was nerve-wracking to be away from my baby for 4 hours, but it was incredibly rewarding and healing to walk into a theater in downtown Los Angeles and see something I had created on the big screen.

To me, self-care is doing something that feeds your soul. It's not worrying about whether others think you're selfish, crazy, or self-consumed. It's about honoring your gifts, taking deep breaths, and reminding yourself, "I am proud of you. Keep shining."

Since then, I've continued my artistry. I've directed more projects and even created an Artist Wellness Day, which has been one of the most incredible experiences I've shared with people I love and admire. So, here's a little token of encouragement: whatever burns deep inside you to create or pursue, don't give up on it. It may take a little longer—just like the book I'm currently writing—but keep manifesting the life you envision for yourself. Keep going.

Because self-care isn't optional—it's essential. I love spa days but it's not just about that. It's about survival and balance. Without it, exhaustion and stress can leave you feeling like you're running on empty, unable to care for yourself or your baby the way you want to. As a new mom, your body is healing, your hormones are shifting, and your mind is stretched in ways you've never experienced before. Self-care helps you recharge, rebuild, and meet the challenges of motherhood with strength and resilience.

In this chapter, we'll explore self-care and mindfulness practices tailored for new moms. You'll learn how to identify what you truly need, create realistic routines, and incorporate small but meaningful moments into your busy days. Self-care isn't about doing it all—it's about doing what matters most for your well-being so you can be the best version of a mom. Let's start by looking at why putting yourself first is one of the best gifts you can give your baby.

8.1 MINDFULNESS EXERCISES FOR THE MOM ON THE GO

Picture this: you're standing in the kitchen, washing bottles, your mind racing with a never-ending to-do list, and the baby's cries in the background. Sound familiar? It's in moments like these that mindfulness can be a game-changer. Contrary to popular belief, mindfulness isn't just for yogis or monks; it's for anyone looking to create a little calm oasis.

Mindfulness simply means being present—focusing on the here and now instead of getting lost in the noise of daily life. Studies show it can lower stress by easing your mind and reducing cortisol levels. With regular practice, it helps you react thoughtfully rather than impulsively, making even the toughest moments feel a little more manageable.

Easy Mindfulness Habits to Try

Incorporating mindfulness doesn't require hours of free time (because let's face it, who has that?). Here are some quick, practical exercises to fit into your day:

- **Morning Breathing:** Start your day with a five-minute breathing session. Find a quiet space, close your eyes, and take slow, deep breaths. Feel the air fill your lungs and flow out. And it can be done in bed, even before you start your day.
- **Mindful Eating:** During meals, put distractions aside. Savor each bite. It's a simple way to slow down and turn eating into a mini meditation.
- **Body Scan Before Bed:** As you wind down, lie comfortably and mentally check in with your body. From your head to your toes, notice any tension and let it go. This practice helps you release the day's stress and prepare for better sleep.
- **Cut some cords** before bed or at any part of the day; briefly envision all the interactions of the day, all the things you have seen online or on tv, or the people you drove on the road with, envision small cords attached to your heart connecting you to everything you have encountered, envision a scissor cutting these cords, see the cord fall to the floor, dispersing into dust, send everyone and yourself some love. Think of it as an emotional reset.

Bringing Mindfulness into Parenting

Mindfulness isn't just about self-care; it can also deepen your connection with your child. For example:

- **Active Listening:** Give your little one your full attention during conversations. Listen without distractions and respond with care—this strengthens your bond and supports their emotional growth.
- **Playtime with Presence:** Whether stacking blocks or playing in the park, engage fully in the activity. No phones, no multitasking—just you and your child, making memories in the moment.

If you need a little help getting started, there are plenty of resources to guide you. Apps like Calm and Headspace provide quick, guided meditations that fit perfectly into busy schedules. If you prefer reading, books like *The Mindful Parent* by Amber Hatch offer practical advice on how to bring mindfulness into family life. My favorite author is Louise Hay, and her book "Affirmations to Heal Your Life" is one of the most life-altering books for me. I loved reading a page about mindset shifts and incorporating these new thought patterns into my life. Online communities can also be a great source of support—joining forums or groups where other parents share mindfulness tips, challenges, and successes can make the journey feel less lonely.

It's all about finding small moments of peace in your hectic day. By slowing down, focusing on the present, and letting go of judgment, you can create space to enjoy life's little joys—whether it's a single breath, a bite of food, or the sight of a block tower being built by tiny hands.

8.2 SPEEDY SWEAT SESSIONS FOR BUSY NEW MOMS

After a busy day, squeezing in a workout might feel tough, but it's worth it. Exercise isn't just about getting back to your pre-pregnancy body—it's about boosting your energy, improving your mood, and carving out time for yourself. Even a short burst of activity can help you feel refreshed and clear your mind, like hitting a reset button for both your body and mental health. Regular movement not only strengthens your muscles and posture but also supports your overall well-being.

You don't need a gym or fancy equipment to get started. Just ten minutes can make a difference. Grab a couple of soup cans to use as weights for a quick home workout—try some squats, lunges, or arm curls without even leaving your living room.

Prefer something gentler? Postpartum-friendly yoga stretches like cat-cow or simple twists can help regain flexibility while soothing your body. And for cardio, get creative with what's around you. A brisk stroll with your baby in the stroller or a kitchen dance break to your favorite playlist can boost your heart rate and flood your body with feel-good endorphins. Trust me, a two-song dance session can completely shift your energy.

Of course, safety comes first, especially during the postpartum phase. Many new moms worry about core issues like diastasis recti (The separation of abdominal muscles). The key here is to focus on exercises that promote recovery, like pelvic tilts or heel slides, which build strength gently. For those dealing with loose joints from hormone changes, opt for low-impact movements like walking instead of running to keep your body protected while staying active.

It's also important to keep your goals realistic. This isn't about drastic changes or running a race next month; it's about celebrating the small wins. You can start a fitness journal to track progress—note when you fit in a walk, a stretch, or a bit of strength training. Each entry becomes proof of your determination. Maybe today you notice a little more stamina or feel a bit more flexible—acknowledge those moments. They're meaningful steps on your journey toward feeling strong and empowered.

And for a little extra motivation, try using a simple fitness tracker. Write down your goals for the week, check off what you've accomplished, and reflect on how each session makes you feel. Seeing your progress builds momentum and reminds you of your incredible resilience.

Motherhood comes with endless demands, and it's easy to put your needs last. But movement is your secret ally, a way to recharge, strengthen, and care for yourself—not just physically, but in every way. You deserve this time, and your body and mind will thank you for it.

8.3 PEN YOUR WAY TO PROGRESS

Journaling can feel like having a trusted friend—one who listens, keeps your secrets, and never judges. But what about privacy? There's always a chance someone could read your thoughts. If that worries you, you can always revisit and rip up pages later. Journaling is for you, so write freely, knowing you can decide what stays or goes.

It's no surprise that studies show journaling can reduce stress and improve emotional well-being, with nearly 15% of adults turning to it as a form of self-care. For new moms, it can be especially powerful—a personal space to pour out emotions, process the whirlwind of motherhood, and find some clarity.

Motherhood brings an overwhelming mix of joy, exhaustion, love, and self-discovery. Journaling is not just writing on a page; it's creating a safe space to explore your emotions, rediscover your identity, and celebrate the victories—big or small—along the way. As you jot down your thoughts, you might uncover patterns, gain new perspectives, or simply feel a weight lifted. It's a moment of calm in a busy day, a gentle reminder that your feelings matter, too.

If you're unsure where to start, prompts can be a helpful guide. Write about the highlights of your day or the challenges you've faced as a new mom. What made you smile? What tested your patience? Reflect on how motherhood has reshaped your identity—what's changed, and what parts of you remain the same? Consider setting intentions or goals for yourself, both as a mother and an individual. These small steps can offer clarity, helping you feel grounded as you navigate this new chapter.

And remember, journaling doesn't have to be all words. Let your creativity flow. Sketch, doodle, or pair your thoughts with drawings —it's a freeing way to express yourself when words don't feel enough. Or try creating a vision board—cut out images and words that represent your dreams and aspirations, crafting a tangible reminder of what you're striving for. These creative layers can make the experience even more meaningful.

Pro tip: when creating a vision board, include pictures of things that have come true in your life as proof to the world/ universe that you have created/manifested wonderful things.

Take Patricia, for example. As a new mom feeling swamped by the demands of motherhood, she began a nightly journaling routine. Over time, she noticed recurring emotions and thoughts that helped her better understand her needs. Journaling became her sanctuary, rekindling passions she'd set aside and giving her a renewed sense of purpose. Then there's Emily, who started journaling daily affirmations of gratitude. Focusing on the positives—not just the stressors— helped her feel lighter, more resilient, and ready to face challenges with optimism. These stories are a testament to how journaling can transform not only your outlook but also your journey through motherhood.

As you embrace the beautiful, messy, and ever-changing world of motherhood, let your journal be your ally. With each entry, you are letting yourself choose peace, self-care, and progress. And as your child grows, you'll have a treasured record of your own growth alongside them.

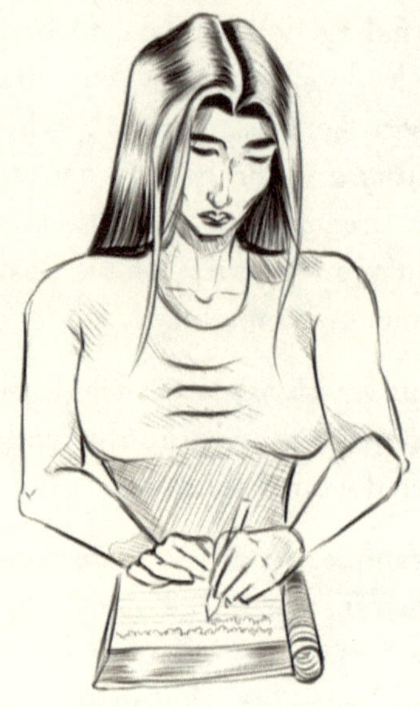

SELF-CARE REFLECTION EXERCISE

Take a moment to reflect and integrate self-care into your daily routine. This simple exercise will help you focus on the positive aspects of your life and the support systems that keep you grounded. Grab a notebook and write down the following:

1. **Three Activities That Bring You Joy**

Think about simple things that make you happy. Examples: enjoying a skincare routine, sipping coffee or tea, reading a book, taking an uninterrupted bath, going for a 15-minute walk alone, getting a massage, brushing your hair, lifting weights, meeting a friend for lunch, meditating at a beautiful location, or even dressing up for the day.

____

____

2. Two People Who Support You

Who are the people that uplift your spirits and give you strength? Examples: your husband, best friend, cousin, neighbor, co-worker, therapist, mom, sister, or anyone in your support network.

____

____

3. One Thing You're Grateful For

Reflect on something in your life you truly appreciate. Examples: your comfy bed, your safe home, the food in your fridge, the ability to walk around freely, your healthy body, your baby's health, or having a reliable car.

____

____

Do this exercise daily to center yourself and remind yourself of the joy, support, and gratitude in your life — even during challenging times. Self-care is essential for your well-being, giving you the strength to navigate the complexities of life and motherhood.

CHAPTER 9
A HOLISTIC GUIDE TO POSTPARTUM BLISS

During one of my shifts, I cared for a mother from a culture deeply rooted in community rituals and traditions. After the birth of her first child, her extended family came together in the days following her delivery, bringing with them foods prepared with traditional herbs believed to promote recovery and lactation. They had a designated family member who would massage the mother's body daily with warm oils and another who would take care of household tasks to allow the new mother to rest and bond with her baby.

This experience reinforced my passion about the connection between food, culture, and care—a theme that has resonated deeply in my own life. I myself, have been vegetarian since 2007. I read a book called Skinny Bitch, and it converted me to a plant-based lifestyle—I have never looked back. Anyone who knows me knows how much I love going to the farmer's market. Since 2011, I have made it my mission to experience the colorful bliss of connecting with farmers, eating seasonal vegetables, and asking, "What the heck is that?" Then I ask them how to cook it and learn all about the yummy food planet Earth has to offer. I strongly believe in the power of food to not only nourish our bodies but also connect us to our roots and cultural traditions.

The postpartum period is a time of significant change and adjustment, both physically and emotionally, for new mothers. While attention is often focused on the newborn, a mother's well-being is equally critical during this stage. This chapter explores holistic approaches to postpartum care, emphasizing the importance of addressing physical recovery, mental health, and emotional support. By integrating diverse strategies such as proper nutrition, mindfulness practices, and community support, this chapter aims to provide a comprehensive guide to fostering a balanced and healthy postpartum experience.

9.1 THE POSTPARTUM PLATE

The kitchen, often the heart of the home, can be a place of healing after having a baby. I remember a mom, Mia, telling me how much comfort she found in her morning routine of making a green smoothie. As the blender whirred, she'd tell herself she was strong and healthy. That simple habit reminded her to take care of herself, not just for her, but for her baby too.

The postpartum period is a critical time for a new mother's physical and emotional well-being. During this time, the body has gone through significant changes and needs proper nourishment to support healing and recovery. The demands of caring for a newborn can also be physically exhausting, making it crucial for mothers to maintain good nutrition to keep up with their energy levels.

Studies show that proper nutrition during the postpartum period can significantly impact a mother's recovery and overall health. According to the World Health Organization (WHO), iron deficiency anemia, which affects up to 30% of postpartum women globally, can be mitigated with a diet rich in iron and vitamin C. Additionally, research from the Journal of Perinatal Education highlights that 75% of breastfeeding mothers require an additional 450–500 calories per day to support milk production.

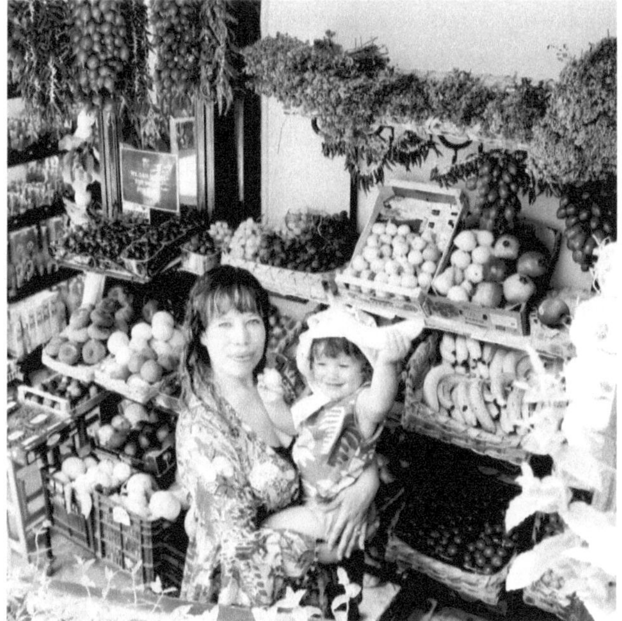

Me and Nikola — June 23, 2024 Positano, Italy | Photo by Eric Dilauro I love teaching every baby I've ever loved how magical food can be—the scent of ripe peaches, the soft curve of a banana, the bright zest of a lemon held in tiny hands. We visit farmer's markets to explore it all—touching, smelling, tasting, learning. Here we are in one of my favorite places on earth, sun on our skin, fruit in hand, hearts wide open.

Therefore, maintaining a balanced and nutrient-dense diet can not only benefit the mother but also her breastfeeding baby. This chapter focuses on the power of good nutrition and how it can support recovery after childbirth.

There is an old saying, "Let food be thy medicine and medicine be thy food." It's a time-tested approach to healing, especially during the postpartum period. Nutrient-dense foods play a critical role in recovery, helping to repair tissues, reduce inflammation, and provide the energy needed to care for your newborn. Think leafy greens, berries, lean proteins, and omega-3-rich ingredients like walnuts, chia seeds, and olive oil. These foods fuel your body's restoration while supporting emotional well-being and brain health.

Anti-inflammatory diets are particularly powerful for postpartum recovery. Foods like turmeric (rich in curcumin), spirulina, and Brussels sprouts help reduce inflammation and ease discomfort. A sprinkle of turmeric in your meals or tea can go a long way in supporting your healing process. Incorporating these simple adjustments can soothe both body and mind.

Essential nutrients like iron, omega-3 fatty acids, and probiotics are key for postpartum health. Iron-rich foods like spinach, lentils, and quinoa combat fatigue and replenish energy after childbirth. Omega-3s, found in flaxseeds and edamame, support cognitive function and emotional balance, benefiting both you and your baby if breastfeeding. Probiotics in yogurt and fermented foods like sauerkraut strengthen your gut health, boosting nutrient absorption and immunity.

Meal planning can simplify postpartum nutrition. Batch-cook hearty soups, stews, or casseroles that are easy to reheat, ensuring you have balanced meals even when life gets wild. Aim for plates with lean protein, whole grains, and colorful vegetables to cover all your nutrient needs. For quick fixes, smoothies are a lifesaver—try blending spinach, banana, almond milk, and protein powder for a vibrant, nutrient-packed start to your day. Or whip up a simple veggie soup with quinoa and herbs for a comforting, protein-rich meal. With the right foods, you can nourish your body, ease recovery, and thrive during this transformative time.

I loved walking around with my huge pregnant belly and, the following week postpartum, having my newborn baby in my Artipoppe pouch, twirling in my dress, and finally living out my vision of my baby joining me at the farmers market. Now, as a toddler, Nikola picks out his fruits and lets the farmers know when he is ready to pay.

That being said—I may not be body-right, body-tight right now, but I am someone who chooses healthy, vibrant foods 80% of the time. So, if you're far from being a super healthy eater, start with choosing to be open to colorful, non-processed foods. Add different seasonings, go to markets, and just ask how people cook things. Purchase at least one thing and make it with love and intention, knowing you are nourishing your body with food freshly picked off the tree.

Equally important to nourishing your body with the right foods is taking time to nurture your mind and spirit. Incorporating practices like yoga and meditation into your routine can provide balance and support overall well-being during any phase of life.

9.2 RECONNECTING TO YOUR ZEN THROUGH YOGA & MEDITATION

Motherhood is fast-paced and overwhelming. In the midst of sleepless nights and endless to-do lists, finding moments of calm can feel impossible. Yet, incorporating yoga and meditation into your routine can be a transformative tool for postpartum recovery—emotionally and physically. Studies show that mindfulness practices like yoga can reduce postpartum depression symptoms by up to 40%, proving their power to support new moms in transitioning to this life-changing role. I have listed what I have seen work wonders for myself and many other mothers.

Yoga is more than just physical exercise—it helps your mind and body. Postpartum poses like cat-cow stretches and twists can reduce back and shoulder tension from nursing and holding your baby. These movements also help rebuild core strength and flexibility as you recover after childbirth. Just 10 minutes on the mat at home can bring some calm to your day.

Breathing techniques, or pranayama, are a hidden gem of yoga that you can use anytime, anywhere. Slow, intentional breaths calm your nervous system, reduce stress, and bring clarity to a busy mind. Try this: breathe in and out through your nose, inhale deeply for four counts, hold for four, then exhale for six. With each breath, let go of tension and invite calm. These simple exercises act as a quick "reset" button during overwhelming moments.

Meditation is another powerful tool for new moms. It promotes mindfulness—a state of focused awareness that helps you stay present and emotionally balanced. Guided meditations are an easy way to begin, offering structure and support as you ease into the practice. Gratitude meditation, for instance, shifts your focus from stress to appreciation. Close your eyes and think of three things you're grateful for—small or big. This brief moment of reflection can brighten your mood and reduce anxiety.

If yoga and meditation feel intimidating, start small and tailor these practices to your needs. Gentle yoga styles like Hatha or restorative yoga are perfect for easing back into movement. Create a simple meditation space at home, even if it's just a corner with a cushion. Add calming elements like soft lighting or your favorite scent to make it inviting.

The key is consistency, not perfection.

For a fresh twist on mindfulness, consider adding activities like dancing or tapping (EFT) to your toolkit. A quick dance session to your favorite song can lift your spirits and energize your body. Tapping, which involves gently tapping acupressure points while focusing on stress, helps release emotional blocks and promotes relaxation. Both are great ways to reconnect with your body and emotions in a fun, accessible way.

Plenty of resources can help you get started. Apps like YogaGlo and Headspace offer guided yoga and meditation sessions designed for new mothers, while online classes let you practice at your own pace. Books like *The First Forty Days* and *The Mindful Mom-To-Be* provide insightful exercises and tips to deepen your mindfulness journey. These tools make it easier to prioritize your well-being, even in your busiest moments.

With these practices in mind, nurturing your overall well-being becomes a manageable and rewarding part of your routine. Now that we know more about how to practice mindfulness, let's think about how to get our creative spark back.

9.3 THE HEALING POWER OF ART & PLAY

You know what life after birth feels like? It can feel like your days start with assessing the texture of poop and end with looking to see if the bum redness has gone away. However, being a mother doesn't mean giving up on your passions and creative pursuits. In fact, it may be more crucial than ever to make time for them as an outlet for stress and self-expression.

It provides a therapeutic outlet for stress and emotional release, helping mothers navigate the complex swirl of emotions that often accompany this phase of life. Motherhood has a way of surfacing feelings—some joyful, others deeply challenging. Channeling those emotions into creative projects can offer a sense of calm like no other.

Engaging in art allows emotions to take shape visually, bypassing the limits of words. Painting, drawing, or crafting creates a space where feelings can be explored safely, transforming them into something tangible. The rhythmic act of creating—whether it's the flow of a paintbrush or the assembly of a collage—can soothe the mind and uplift the spirit. It's less about producing a masterpiece and more about immersing yourself in the process, finding peace in the act of making.

For example, painting or sketching provides a meditative escape. You don't need fancy supplies—just watercolors, pencils, or even recycled materials like old magazines or leaves. Crafting, especially with sustainable materials, can be both grounding and rewarding. Similarly, combining journaling with visual elements like doodles or collages offers a unique way to process emotions, blending words and imagery to reflect your inner world.

Art also has a magical way of fostering connection. Joining a local art class or workshop can introduce you to a community of mothers who share similar experiences. These gatherings create a support network where stories, advice, and laughter flow as freely as creativity. Melissa, a mother recovering from postpartum depression, found a local art workshop to be her lifeline, offering her a sense of belonging while reigniting her spark for life. Emma, another mom, turned to painting during postpartum and described it as a release — each brushstroke helping her process her emotions and find clarity.

The healing power of creativity lies in its ability to turn pain, cluttered thoughts, or even joy into something meaningful. It's a reminder that recovery doesn't have to be linear or conventional; it can be vibrant, messy, and deeply personal.

Next, we'll explore the importance of building your own community and finding support during the postpartum period.

9.4 BUILDING YOUR MOM TRIBE

Imagine sitting in your living room, baby in your arms, surrounded by a group of mothers who truly understand what you're going through. They know the late-night feedings, the endless diaper changes, and the sheer exhaustion. This is the power of a mom tribe —a community that offers more than just companionship. It provides emotional support and shared experiences that can greatly improve your postpartum well-being. Being part of a supportive group reminds you that you're not alone. Sharing advice, laughing over parenting mishaps, and celebrating milestones together creates a unique and meaningful bond. These connections can ease feelings of isolation and replace them with a sense of belonging and understanding.

As someone who is surrounded by new moms on the daily, I still had a tough time building my own tribe. At first, I thought that because I saw it so much, I knew what postpartum loneliness looked like, and that knowledge would somehow protect me from the worst of it. Boy, was I wrong! It wasn't until I actively sought out and joined various mom groups that I truly understood the value of having a supportive community during this time.

Building your own mom tribe might feel intimidating, but it's a rewarding process. Here are some steps you can take to find your support system:

- Join local parenting groups or classes to meet moms in similar stages of motherhood.
- Search for local mom groups at the park for music classes, and mommy & me classes.
- Check out your local library and see what classes they offer.
- Look into your free community led classes, see what types of activities are offered at your neighborhood churches.
- See if your local community center has free or low-cost activities available.
- Explore social media communities tailored to different parenting styles and interests.
- Participate in online forums or groups to connect with moms from home.
- Gain advice and support from digital mom tribes, offering a safe space to share struggles and triumphs.
- Benefit from peer support, which provides understanding, tips, and fresh solutions.
- Organize play dates or group activities for socialization and bonding for both moms and babies.
- Create special memories by watching your baby interact with others while connecting with fellow moms.
- Engage in community-led initiatives, such as meal trains, childcare swaps, or wellness workshops, to foster unity and support.

Building a mom tribe is about more than making friends—it's about creating a support system that enhances your life and well-being. The connections you make can provide comfort during tough times and bring even more joy to motherhood. As you continue your journey, embrace the strength of community and the value of shared experiences. In the next chapter, we'll look at global postpartum care practices and the role of extended family in supporting new moms.

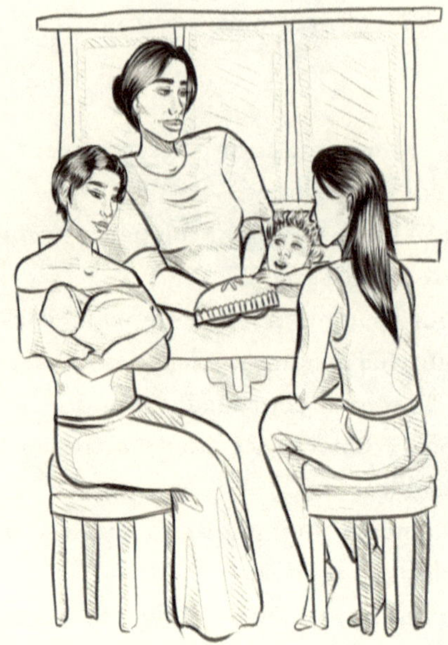

Exercise: Finding Your Mom Tribe

Step 1: Research Different Mom Groups

- List three ways you will search for mom communities (e.g., local meetups, social media groups, parenting classes, neighborhood events).
- Identify what kind of support you are looking for (e.g., emotional support, parenting tips, playdates).

____

____

____

Step 2: Attend & Observe

- Choose one or two groups to explore first.
- Pay attention to how you feel in the group—do you feel comfortable, heard, and supported?

____

____

____

Step 3: Keep an Open Mind

- Remember: Not every mom in a group will be your match, and that's okay!
- Finding your mom tribe is like dating—you may not click with everyone, but you will find at least one person who sparks joy and makes parenting more enjoyable.

____

____

____

Step 4: Reflect & Adjust

- After attending a few gatherings, journal your thoughts:
    - Did you feel a sense of connection?
    - What worked for you? What didn't?
    - Do you want to try a different group or go deeper into one you liked?

____

____

____

Your mom tribe doesn't have to be big—it just needs to include people who uplift and support you. Also, you may not necessarily resonate with all the moms of the group. It's similar to high school sometimes. But you will find at least one person that will bring you so much joy that it will make parenting more enjoyable for you. Just keep exploring until you find the connections that feel right for you.

CHAPTER 10
GLOBAL PERSPECTIVES ON POSTPARTUM CARE

I'm probably the proudest Dominican you'll ever meet—though my cousin Angie jokes it's because I wasn't actually born there. Still, I carry so much pride for my roots, for the beauty of my people, and for their passion for love, music, and joy.

I love how my culture moves its hips and sings with eyes closed, completely lost in the rhythm. I love breaking a deep sweat dancing bachata and merengue, feeling every note in my bones.

This is why I want my baby to fall in love with his culture, too—all of it. The Dominican, Italian, and French-Canadian blood that flows through his veins. He's already traveled to each of his ancestral lands, and if you have the privilege of returning to the land of your parents, I encourage you to do the same. Reignite that cultural passion in your children. Let them feel it, live it, and carry it forward.

I always remind my friends: *Every baby is their own unique human, and every mother was an individual person long before she became a parent.* No two postpartum journeys are the same. Each experience is shaped by who we are, what we value, and the lives we lived before motherhood.

Yet, across the world, you'll find cultural traditions that offer shared wisdom about healing, nurturing, and community support after birth. From ancient rituals passed down through generations to modern medical care, postpartum practices weave together health, family, and a deep reverence for new life.

In this chapter, we'll explore diverse postpartum traditions around the globe—and how cultural values and community resources shape a mother's healing journey, influence infant outcomes, and remind us that while every story is unique, none of us are meant to walk this path alone.

10.1 CULTURAL INFLUENCES ON POSTPARTUM CARE

In many cultures, postpartum care is deeply rooted in cultural beliefs and practices that have been passed down through generations. These traditions often center around the concept of "confinement," or a period of rest and recovery after childbirth. Traveling the world has always been a source of fascination for me since childhood. Each destination offers a chance to deepen understanding and compassion for others. Observing how people spend their days—whether at the park or during quiet moments on public transportation—brings so much joy. Watching families play, laugh, and share meals together is one of life's simple pleasures. My dream is to explore the world with my baby, sharing with him the beauty of diverse perspectives and experiences. But there is no doubt that postpartum care in each culture varies significantly.

In Chinese culture, for example, it is common for new mothers to follow a strict confinement period known as "zuò yuè zi" (坐月子), which translates to "sitting the month." This tradition involves staying indoors, avoiding cold foods and drinks, and being cared for by family members.

Postpartum care traditions around the world emphasize rest, nourishment, and recovery, offering valuable insights into how different cultures support new mothers.

In Korea, "Samchilil" highlights rest and nourishing foods, with specialized care centers, known as "sanhujoriwon," providing tailored recovery support. Similarly, India's Ayurvedic approach focuses on restoring the mother's body through a holistic blend of warm, nutrient-rich foods like ghee and lentils, daily massages with herbal oils, and herbal treatments to promote healing and reduce stress.

In various African cultures, such as Nigeria's "Omugwo" tradition, postpartum care is rooted in community support. Mothers or mothers-in-law provide rest, nourishment, and practical help, enabling the new mother to bond with her baby and recover. In Europe, Germany's "Wochenbett" and the Netherlands' "kraamzorg" place emphasis on professional support, with midwives or caregivers visiting mothers at home to assist with recovery and baby care. Across Latin America, the "cuarentena" offers a 40-day period of rest and a restorative diet, while in Japan, traditions like "satogaeri bunben" involve returning to the family home for support and connection.

Despite cultural differences, there are many common themes—rest, proper nutrition, and community involvement are universal pillars of postpartum recovery. Maternal diets often feature nutrient-dense foods to promote healing, lactation, and energy replenishment, while traditions encourage bonding, emotional well-being, and physical recovery.

These practices offer ideas for improving postpartum care. Simple steps like drinking calming herbal teas, such as ginger or chamomile, or doing gentle postpartum exercises like yoga or traditional dance, can support recovery and well-being. Exploring these cultural perspectives helps us understand how community and tradition shape the postpartum experience, highlighting the universal importance of care during this time.

10.2 THE ROLE OF EXTENDED FAMILY IN DIFFERENT CULTURES

Imagine your grandmother, her hands gently guiding yours as you cradle your newborn. In many cultures, this scenario is part of a cherished tradition where extended family plays a vital role in postpartum care. Grandparents, especially grandmothers, often step in as caregivers, offering the kind of emotional and practical support that only comes with years of experience. If you ask me, the biggest flex of all time is having grandparents nearby to support you during the postpartum period. Their presence can help ease the transition into parenthood, acting as a buffer against the sleepless nights and new responsibilities. In households or cultures where grandparents live nearby—or even in the same home—the postpartum period can feel more manageable, surrounded by the wisdom and steadiness they provide.

However, not everyone has the privilege of having grandparents available or healthy enough to help during this critical time. Often, many of us find ourselves caring for aging family members while also navigating parenthood.

This dual responsibility, often referred to as the "sandwich generation" struggle, can place a significant emotional and physical strain on individuals. Caring for aging parents comes with its own set of challenges, such as managing medical appointments, handling financial concerns, and addressing the emotional toll of watching loved ones lose independence. Adding a newborn to the equation amplifies the pressures, as new parents are already overwhelmed with sleepless nights, constant feedings, and learning to meet the demands of a baby. The combination can lead to feelings of exhaustion, stress, and even guilt, as time and energy inevitably feel stretched too thin.

In these cases, support might come from another elder, a trusted family member, or even a close friend who steps into that nurturing role.

Beyond grandparents, other family members also play a key role in raising children. Aunts and uncles often step in as secondary caregivers, offering everything from help with daily tasks to emotional support. In close-knit families, their involvement fosters a sense of community, creating a strong network that surrounds new parents with love and assistance. Siblings, too, can contribute in unique ways

—older children can lend a hand with younger ones, fostering bonds and a sense of responsibility that strengthen family ties.

Cultural norms heavily influence the role of extended family in childcare. In some communities, new mothers are expected to return to their parents' home after giving birth, allowing the extended family to take on a significant caregiving role. This tradition provides both physical help and emotional reassurance, creating a nurturing environment for recovery. However, these practices aren't without challenges. In cultures where familial duties are emphasized, there may be pressure to conform to traditional roles, which might clash with personal preferences or modern lifestyles. Navigating these expectations often requires finding a balance between respecting tradition and maintaining individuality.

Take, for example, a family living in a multigenerational household. While the constant support can be a blessing, it may also lead to conflicts over parenting styles or lifestyle differences. A grandmother may offer traditional remedies, while the mother incorporates modern parenting techniques. These moments can create opportunities for shared learning, blending different approaches to caregiving and enriching the family dynamic. However, they also underscore the need for clear communication and mutual respect to ensure harmony.

For some, close-knit family structures provide the benefits of a strong support network and a deep sense of belonging. Yet, they can also present challenges, such as blurred boundaries or a lack of personal space. Managing these dynamics requires open conversations and setting clear expectations. It might involve discussing responsibilities, addressing differences in parenting approaches, or simply carving out time for your own family unit. Balancing family traditions with personal preferences can be tricky, but it's essential for maintaining healthy relationships.

So, how can you navigate family involvement in a way that feels supportive rather than overwhelming? Start by setting clear lines of communication. Share your vision for postpartum care with your family and discuss how they can support you in meaningful ways. Be honest about your boundaries, whether it's requesting help with specific tasks, needing alone time, or addressing differences in child-care approaches. Remember, it's okay to say no to offers that don't align with your needs, and it's equally okay to ask for help when you need it.

Approaching these relationships with empathy and clarity can transform the postpartum experience into one where love and care from your extended family truly enhance your journey into parenthood. With the right balance, your family's involvement can provide both the support you need and the space to embrace your own parenting style.

10.3 OLD-SCHOOL WISDOM MEETS MODERN POSTPARTUM HACKS

In today's world, new mothers navigate a mix of timeless postpartum wisdom and modern healthcare tools. It's about finding balance—like sipping fenugreek tea for its lactation benefits while updating your feeding app or joining an online support group session. Integrating these elements creates a well-rounded postpartum care experience.

This balance goes beyond physical recovery, blending ancestral wisdom with modern parenting philosophies. Practices like using healing herbs are gaining renewed attention, especially when backed by scientific research. These traditions help mothers connect with their roots, while modern parenting encourages flexibility, allowing them to choose what works best for their individual situations.

The benefits of this approach are notable. Physically, combining herbal remedies with modern treatments can aid recovery by easing sore muscles, boosting milk production, and lifting mood. Emotionally, it builds a sense of connection by merging traditional practices with modern support networks, offering a variety of resources. This dual approach enhances overall well-being and provides mothers with a versatile set of tools for postpartum care.

Take Ana, for instance. She learned about healing herbs from her grandmother. As a new mom, she worked with both a healthcare provider and an herbalist to create a postpartum plan. This included relaxing herbal infusions and energy-boosting supplements recommended by her doctor. This combination helped her recover efficiently. Similarly, Leah combined cultural traditions with her modern routine by attending yoga classes and embracing postpartum massage rituals, creating a routine that supported both her body and mind.

Successfully blending these practices requires cultural sensitivity and respect. Understanding the origins of traditional methods ensures they're used thoughtfully. Collaborating with herbalists, traditional healers, and healthcare providers helps create informed plans that complement modern treatments. The goal is to develop a balanced approach that prioritizes the mother's health and well-being.

This process is about discovery and personalization. By combining traditional and modern practices, mothers can craft a postpartum experience that feels both supportive and meaningful. It's a way to honor the wisdom of the past while benefiting from modern advancements, creating a postpartum journey that balances tradition and innovation.

10.4 LEARNING FROM DIFFERENT PARENTING STYLES

One of the most frequent concerns I have seen among mothers after birth is the 'what now?' feeling. It's a natural instinct to question whether you are doing things right or not, and in many cases, it leads to comparing your parenting style with others.

But here's the thing: Parenting styles around the world are as diverse as the cultures they come from. From attachment parenting to authoritative parenting, there are various approaches that parents take in raising their children. Each style may have its own benefits and challenges, but learning from different parenting styles can provide valuable insights for new mothers.

One common thread among all these styles is the importance placed on the well-being of the child. Whether it's through gentle or strict methods, parents ultimately want what's best for their child. While some cultures may prioritize independence and self-sufficiency, others may focus on community and interdependence. Let's look at some of the parenting styles around the world.

Parenting Styles Around the World

In some indigenous communities, attachment parenting is common. Babies are carried close, with their needs met immediately and warmly. This closeness creates a strong bond early on, supported by the wisdom of elders who guide younger generations. In these societies, children are never alone, always surrounded by the rhythm of life and connection. This approach emphasizes building a secure foundation for children to grow confidently.

In many African cultures, parenting is a communal effort where the phrase "it takes a village" truly comes to life. Raising children is a shared responsibility, involving parents, elders, and even young peers who contribute companionship. This collective system ensures parents are supported, and children benefit from diverse guidance. It fosters a strong sense of belonging and shared responsibility, creating a nurturing and supportive environment.

In Japan, parenting focuses on fostering unity and mutual respect. From an early age, children are taught the importance of collaboration and social harmony. The concept of *amae* encourages children to rely on caregivers, while also teaching independence and responsibility through daily tasks like chores. This balance of support and autonomy shapes both family life and children's ability to integrate into society.

In India, parenting is deeply connected to family loyalty, education, and cultural traditions. Respect for elders and a focus on academic success are emphasized. Stories, rituals, and celebrations play a key role in teaching values and strengthening family bonds. Indian parenting combines warmth with structure, helping children develop self-discipline and a strong sense of cultural identity.

In Latin America, parenting focuses on warmth, affection, and family closeness. Extended families play a key role in raising children and creating a strong support system. Family meals are a central part of daily life, providing opportunities to bond, share, and pass on values. This approach fosters emotional resilience and lifelong family connections built on compassion and respect.

Growing up in a lively Latino household, my own experience was filled with music, the aroma of home-cooked food, and constant laughter. Our home was always bustling with extended family members. Respect for elders was a core value, and disagreeing openly wasn't encouraged. Despite the strict rules, the environment was full of unconditional love and warmth, creating a childhood rich with joyful memories.

In Scandinavian countries like Sweden, Denmark, and Norway, parenting takes a different approach, emphasizing independence and autonomy from an early age. Children are encouraged to learn through exploration and experience, building self-reliance and confidence. Parents act as guides rather than directors, trusting their kids to make choices and learn from the results. This philosophy values freedom and growth, raising children to be both resilient and resourceful.

Modern Parenting Approaches

The Rider Method

In modern times, parenting has evolved to combine traditional practices with newer ideas. One example is the Rider Method, which emphasizes emotional intelligence and critical thinking. In this approach, parents are seen as companions on their children's journey, offering support and guidance rather than strict control. They encourage open dialogue, joint decision-making, and resilience in facing challenges. This method focuses on collaboration, helping children feel valued and heard while learning to solve problems together.

Gentle Parenting

Gentle parenting is another contemporary approach rooted in empathy, respect, and understanding. This style prioritizes emotional connection and avoids punishment-based discipline. Parents practicing gentle parenting often use affirmations like, "I see you're upset. Let's work through this together," fostering trust and mutual respect.

Attachment Parenting

Attachment parenting, inspired by Dr. William Sears, similarly focuses on building secure bonds. Techniques such as co-sleeping, babywearing, and breastfeeding are common, all aimed at creating a foundation of trust and emotional security.

Free-Range Parenting

Free-range parenting emphasizes fostering independence and resilience in children, gaining significant traction for its approach to encouraging children to embrace manageable risks. This practice nurtures a sense of self-reliance and confidence, exemplified by scenarios such as allowing a 10-year-old to navigate the walk to school independently, reinforcing the belief that autonomy cultivates character.

Helicopter Parenting

In stark contrast, helicopter parenting adopts a more involved stance, with parents deeply engaged in nearly every facet of their child's life. Despite facing criticism, this method originates from a profound intention to protect, support, and ensure the well-being of their children.

Parenting philosophies offer a chance to reflect on the values that shape how we nurture our children. Take a moment to reflect on which parenting styles resonate with you. Maybe you're inspired by the emphasis on independence and exploration found in Scandinavian parenting.

There's no one-size-fits-all approach to parenting. Instead, we can combine elements from different philosophies to create a style that fits your family's unique needs. Each parenting approach highlights different aspects of raising children, helping us think about what truly matters and how those values guide our parenting journey.

A mother who practices co-sleeping may find it helps her sleep better and strengthens her bond with her child. Co-sleeping, common in many cultures, values closeness and connection during sleep. Parents in multicultural households also experience the joys and challenges of blending different traditions.

Parenting is all about adaptability—learning from different styles and incorporating what aligns with your values. It encourages us to stay open, try new techniques, and explore approaches that can enhance our parenting journey. By reflecting on our values and goals, we can create a parenting style that feels personal and authentic, honoring both our heritage and future aspirations.

Parenting is a universal experience, expressed in many ways but understood by all. There's no single "right" way to raise a child—only the way that works best for you and your family. This chapter invites you to embrace the diversity of parenting, grow alongside your children, and create a unique approach to care that reflects your family. Remember, your parenting style doesn't need to be fixed—it should evolve as you and your family grow together.

By exploring parenting styles from around the world, we can plant seeds for how we want to raise our children and gain guidance for the postpartum journey. In the next section, we'll focus on practical steps to build resilience and tackle the challenges new mothers face, helping ensure a smoother transition into this transformative phase.

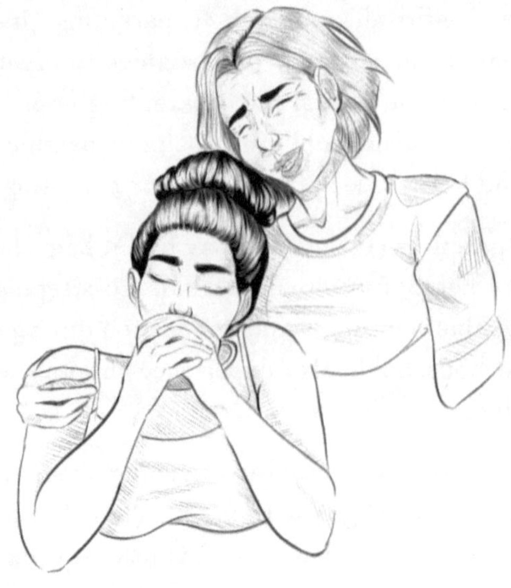

EXERCISE: CRAFTING YOUR PARENTING VALUES

Take a moment to pause and reflect on your personal parenting philosophy. Use the prompts below to explore your values and create a framework for your parenting style:

1. **Reflect on Your Values**
   - What values or principles do you want to emphasize in your parenting?
   - How do these values align with your cultural heritage or your personal beliefs?

   ____

   ____

2. **Learn from Others**
   - Think about a time you admired someone's parenting approach. What specific aspects stood out?

- o Are there international parenting practices you've encountered that resonate with you?

---

3. **Create Your Vision**
   - o Write down three goals you have as a parent.
   - o How do you envision fostering a positive and supportive environment in your family?

---

4. **Practical Steps**
   - o List one new parenting technique you'd like to try in the coming weeks.
   - o Outline how you might address a challenge you're currently facing in your parenting journey.

Use this exercise to connect with your core beliefs, discover inspiration from others, and develop actionable steps toward the parenting approach that feels right for you and your family. Keep your notes as a reminder of your intentions and growth as you move forward!

CHAPTER 11

TURNING CURVEBALLS INTO COMEBACKS

Oh, how life has dramatically changed since the first month of 2025. Our community was devastated starting January 7, 2025, and many of the people we love, care for, and support lost their homes, their farmers' markets, their entire community, and their precious beaches. Our hearts are in deep mourning. Pacific Palisades, Malibu, and Altadena, California, will never be the same.

My heart goes out to our neighbors all around. Our air, our world, our community, and our sense of safety have been forever altered. As we navigate the many changes in this unique moment in time, I want to acknowledge how overwhelming it can all feel—especially when our lives are so deeply intertwined with raising a beam of light, a baby who has chosen to inherit this world.

With so much uncertainty at this moment, I want to remind you that none of us are immune to the changes happening to our planet. I know how overwhelming it can be to raise a baby in these wild times. I don't have the perfect words to say, but I do have a few things that may help.

And I know postpartum life often feels like being hit with a series of curveballs. From adjusting to the new routine, dealing with physical and emotional changes, to trying to navigate through sleepless nights and endless feedings – it can all be overwhelming.

But just like in a baseball game, where curveballs are part of the game, learning how to deal with them is crucial for success. In this chapter, we will discuss ways to handle some challenges and turn them into comebacks.

11.1 THE BEAST THAT IS SLEEP DEPRIVATION

Sleep deprivation is a beast I've wrestled with more times than I can count, and let me tell you, it's a fight that leaves you bruised in more ways than one. The frustration of dragging through the day with a foggy mind and aching body is something I understand deeply. Sleep exhaustion isn't just about being tired; it seeps into every aspect of your life, making even the simplest tasks feel insurmountable. I've stared at the ceiling at 3 a.m., scrolling mindlessly on my phone, convincing myself it's helping me unwind when, in reality, it's stealing the precious hours I so desperately needed to rest.

If there's one thing I've learned, it's that prioritizing sleep isn't just a luxury—it's a necessity. Breaking the cycle of doom scrolling was a game changer for me. I started by setting boundaries with my phone: no screens an hour before bed, and I replaced my late-night scrolling with reading and journaling.

If you're in the trenches of sleep deprivation, my advice is to give yourself grace while taking small, actionable steps. Start with one change, like putting your phone in another room at night or committing to an earlier bedtime a few nights a week. Remember, sleep is foundational to your well-being, and while it may feel elusive during parenting years, it's worth every effort to reclaim. You deserve rest, and your body and mind will thank you for it.

The effects of sleep deprivation are well-known—it can feel like you're navigating life in a fog. Your thoughts get tangled with to-do lists, worries, and an overwhelming longing for sleep. For new parents, sleep deprivation becomes a constant struggle, making even simple tasks like finding your keys or forming a sentence feel exhausting. Cognitive impairment is a common result, and mood swings often follow. One moment, you're irritable, and the next, you're overwhelmed with emotion. Stress and anxiety only add to the problem, creating a cycle where lack of sleep fuels anxiety, and anxiety makes it harder to sleep. This can leave you feeling stuck in survival mode, just trying to get through each day.

But there are ways to get the rest you need. Establishing a consistent bedtime routine can help. Just like you set a routine for your baby, doing the same for yourself can signal your body it's time to wind down. Take a warm bath, spend a few minutes reading or stretching, dim the lights, and avoid screens before bed. Your bedroom should be a calm, restful space. Naps can also be a lifesaver. The advice to "sleep when the baby sleeps" holds true—even short naps can boost your energy and help ease the strain of sleep deprivation. Don't aim for perfection; just focus on getting rest where you can.

Nighttime feedings are another challenge, but being prepared can make them easier. Have bottles, formula, or nursing supplies ready before bed to avoid scrambling in the middle of the night. Personally, I've mastered doing everything in the dark, as even the smallest light can make falling back asleep harder.

Don't hesitate to seek support. Sharing nighttime duties with your partner or family members can make a huge difference. Rotating shifts ensures both of you get some rest. If it's within your budget, a night nurse can be life-changing, providing professional care while you recharge. Having help allows you to get the rest you need to better care for both yourself and your baby.

11.2 DODGING UNSOLICITED PARENTING ADVICE LIKE A PRO

The moment you announce your pregnancy, advice starts pouring in from every direction. It's like joining a club where the price of admission is endless opinions on how to parent. Family members, especially in-laws, often feel the need to share their wisdom. Maybe it's your mother-in-law suggesting an extra blanket for the baby, even in summer, or your father recommending an old-school remedy for a fussy infant.

While these suggestions usually come from a place of love and experience, they can feel like too much or even patronizing at times. Friends, and even strangers, also jump in. The cashier at the grocery store might suggest a sleep trick that worked for her, while your college roommate texts you about the best educational toys. It can feel like everyone is watching your every move, ready to weigh in.

From my own experience, I've learned the best way to deal with unsolicited advice is simple: *acknowledge it, repeat it back, and then stick to your original plan.*

When I first became a parent, I spent a lot of energy explaining my choices to others, especially my family. Each explanation felt exhausting like I had to defend every decision. Sometimes, I even went along with advice I didn't agree with just because I was too tired to argue.

Eventually, I decided to stop. I started treating unsolicited advice like background noise — acknowledging it without letting it weigh on me. If I had the energy, I'd listen, repeat their suggestion back, and thank them. This small change saved me so much energy and gave me a sense of peace. Parenting is hard enough without carrying the weight of everyone else's opinions. Learning to listen but not over-explain became my go-to strategy and allowed me to focus on what really mattered — trusting my own instincts.

Navigating all this advice requires a balance of tact and confidence. One effective approach is politely acknowledging the advice and then steering the conversation elsewhere. A simple "Thank you, I'll think about that" works well to diffuse tension and move on. Humor can also help. If someone insists on a particular method, you might say, "If only babies came with instruction manuals!" to keep things light while still setting boundaries.

Many parents find success by blending tact with practical strategies. Take Lisa, for example. When her mother constantly offered outdated advice, Lisa didn't dismiss it outright. Instead, she found ways to involve her mother in activities that aligned with her parenting style, like preparing meals together or reading with her child. This approach gave her mother a sense of involvement while naturally reducing the flow of unnecessary advice. By focusing on shared, positive experiences, Lisa found a way to keep the peace without compromising her parenting choices.

Another strategy for dealing with unsolicited advice is to redirect the conversation towards a different topic. For instance, if someone starts criticizing your choice to breastfeed, you could steer the conversation towards something else, like asking about their weekend plans or sharing a funny story about your child. This can help shift the focus away from the unwanted advice and keep things light and positive. Or if someone criticizes your use of a pacifier, you could respond with, "This works best for us right now." It's a respectful but firm way to stand by your choices. Remember, your parenting decisions are valid, and you have the right to do what's best for your family.

It's also important to remember that not all advice is bad. Sometimes, even when we don't agree with it, there may be some valuable insights or perspectives that we can gain from hearing others' opinions. It's okay to consider different approaches and decide what works best for you and your family.

However, if someone continues to push their advice despite your attempts to redirect or politely decline, it may be necessary to set boundaries. This can involve firmly stating that you appreciate their concern but are confident in your decisions as a parent. It's also important to communicate that you would prefer not to discuss the topic further.

It's natural for family and friends to want to offer support and guidance, but ultimately, it's up to us as parents to make the best decisions for our children. By using tactful strategies and setting boundaries when needed, we can navigate unsolicited advice while staying true to our own parenting style. Remember, trust yourself and have confidence in your choices - that is what truly matters in raising happy and healthy children.

11.3 LOVING THE SKIN YOU'RE IN

As you go through your pregnancy, your body is being stretched and changed in ways you never imagined. It can be easy to feel self-conscious about your appearance, especially with the societal pressure to "bounce back" quickly after giving birth. But it's important to remember that your body is doing something incredible - growing and nurturing a new life.

Before I got pregnant, I was very fit and proud of my active, healthy lifestyle. I kept that momentum going during my pregnancy, staying active and energized. Despite that, I gained 80 pounds. After delivering my baby, I was shocked and frustrated to see that only 25 pounds came off in the first few weeks. I started counting down the days until I could work out again, believing that returning to my fitness routine would fix everything.

When I finally got the six-week clearance to exercise, I was unmotivated and exhausted. The energy I expected to come rushing back simply wasn't there. Instead of being patient with myself, I became my own worst critic. I constantly compared my postpartum body to how fit and strong I was before. Then, one day, I had a moment of clarity that shifted my perspective.

I realized the harsh way I was speaking to myself mirrored how I used to feel as a 15-year-old struggling with being overweight. That teenage version of me, who needed compassion and support, was now a new mom dealing with breastfeeding, sleep deprivation, and caring for a baby. This was the moment I decided to break the cycle of self-criticism. I promised to approach this stage of my life with kindness and patience.

Instead of obsessing over my pre-baby weight, I focused on small, manageable changes. I drank more water, made healthier food choices, and found time for activities I enjoyed, like spin classes and hot yoga. Slowly, my energy began to return—not because I was pushing myself, but because I was caring for myself. My body hasn't returned to its pre-baby weight yet, and that's okay. I trust my body's ability to recover, but more importantly, I trust myself to continue growing in self-love.

Let's be real - we live in a society that profits from our insecurities, making it all the more important to reject the narrative that our worth is tied to our appearance. For me, postpartum body image has become less about reclaiming my old body and more about embracing the person I am today—a person who is stronger, kinder, and more resilient than ever before.

After giving birth, many of us find ourselves looking in the mirror, facing a body that feels unfamiliar. The pressure to "bounce back" physically can be overwhelming, as if regaining a pre-pregnancy figure is some kind of proof of successful motherhood. It's easy to compare ourselves to magazine covers or social media posts where new moms seem to look flawless just weeks after delivery. But the reality is, those images are often edited and far from the truth. Expecting to immediately lose pregnancy weight and fit back into old jeans is not only unrealistic but unfair. Our bodies have done something incredible, and they need time to heal and change at their own pace.

Building a positive body image begins with self-love and gratitude for the amazing things your body has done—carrying, nourishing, and birthing a child. This doesn't mean forcing yourself to love every stretch mark or extra pound, but rather recognizing the strength and resilience in those features. Each mark and curve are a reminder of growth, perseverance, and love. Surround yourself with positive influences, whether that's friends or media that encourage self-acceptance and celebrate diverse body types. It's much easier to embrace yourself when you're not constantly exposed to narrow and unrealistic beauty standards.

Focusing on health instead of appearance is a powerful shift. Set goals that prioritize feeling strong and energized over a number on the scale. Try activities that make you feel good—like walking, yoga, or dancing around your living room. Celebrate the things your body can do, not just how it looks. Think about the simple joys it brings, like hugging your baby or chasing your toddler. These moments capture the true beauty of motherhood.

Take Belinda's story, for example. She struggled with her body image postpartum, caught in a cycle of self-criticism over what she saw as flaws. But when she joined a local fitness class, her perspective began to change. It wasn't just the exercise — it was the supportive community of women who embraced their bodies at every stage. They encouraged each other, celebrated small victories, and focused on health instead of appearance. Emily's journey toward body confidence wasn't perfect, but it showed the importance of community and self-acceptance.

For others, the path may look different. Shiloh, another mother, found healing through journaling. Writing about her feelings helped her process her emotions and gradually shift her perspective. What she once saw as flaws — like stretch marks or a softer stomach — became symbols of her strength and the life she brought into the world. Her journey shows that self-acceptance can take many forms, and it's about finding what works for you.

Ultimately, creating a positive body image is about embracing imperfection, celebrating your body's strength, and giving yourself the time and grace to heal. Beauty isn't about size or shape — it's about the love and resilience you carry. And remember, you're not alone. There's a community of mothers who understand and support you, each on their own journey toward self-acceptance and empowerment.

11.4 THRIVING WHEN A NEW SIBLING JOINS THE FAMILY

Welcoming a new sibling into the family can be an exciting and challenging time for everyone involved. It is a major transition that requires patience, love, and support from parents and other family members. As a parent, you may worry about how your child will adjust to having a new brother or sister, but there are plenty of tips and tricks to make this transition smoother for everyone. Here are some tips that I found to be helpful.

If possible, mom shouldn't hold the baby the first time the older sibling meets the baby. Acknowledge and check in with the older sibling first, and then, after you've had a moment with them, ask if they are ready to meet the baby.

Make the baby the source of all gifts given to the big brother or big sister. You can say, "The baby wanted you to have this gift," or "The baby wanted you to enjoy a delicious dinner." This way, the baby comes bearing multiple peace offerings to their new household.

Anyone who comes to see the baby should approach the older sibling first and give them some attention before shifting focus to the baby.

If both babies are crying, comfort the older sibling first.

Be mindful of your wording when the older child wants to play or get your attention. Avoid saying things like, "Can't you see I am feeding the baby?" or "I can't right now; the baby needs me." Instead, try repeating back what the older sibling asked for. For example:

- "I would love to play with you. As soon as I'm done feeding the baby, we'll play in 10 minutes. I'm so excited to play with you."
- "Okay, baby, I have to play with big sister, so in 10 minutes, I'm going to put you in your crib so I can play."

Ask the older sibling if they want to help with tasks for the baby, such as getting diapers and wipes.

Express your excitement about having a one-on-one playdate with the older child.

Talk to your child's stuffed animals and tell them how wonderful the child is doing in their new role as big brother or sister.

It's completely normal for the older sibling to experience some regression as they process and try to understand that this new family member is here to stay. So, don't dwell on it for too long.

11.5 RESILIENCE STARTS WITH A GROWTH MINDSET

In early motherhood, resilience is your savior, helping you stay steady through constant changes and uncertainty. Resilience means staying adaptable, finding emotional strength, and maintaining mental toughness despite the challenges. It's about rolling with the punches—whether it's a sudden change in your baby's sleep schedule or dealing with an illness.

Emotional strength helps you stay calm and composed, even on the toughest days and longest nights. Mental toughness gives you the determination to face challenges head-on, knowing you can over-come them. Being resilient doesn't mean you won't feel stressed or overwhelmed—it means you'll have the tools to manage those feelings and keep moving forward. And you can practice resilience just as any other skill by using the following methods.

Every morning, start your day grounded in gratitude. Stay off your phone and take a moment to envision a world where you and your family are safe. Remind your body and mind that you are protected. Stay hydrated, limit screen time, and connect with nature—whatever form that takes for you. Plant something, water something, or simply feel the ground beneath your bare feet. Ground yourself daily, if possible.

Take life one day at a time. Write down your fears and anxieties, but also remind yourself of all the good in your life. Immerse yourself in your community—support local businesses, attend free or low-cost events, and encourage friends and family to come together. There's no better time to build your village of support and connection.

Prepare for the unexpected by putting together an emergency go-bag. Include essentials like original copies of important documents (birth certificates, marriage certificates), some cash, medications, an external charger, and formula if needed. No matter where you live, it's always wise to be ready.

Every day, I remind my child—and myself—that we are safe and protected. I choose to believe in safety, calm, and joy, even in uncertain times. While I know the world is shifting in ways we can't yet fully understand, I focus on what I can control. I know that if my family is together, we will thrive wherever we go, even if we have to start fresh in a new place.

Be patient with yourself and your healing body. Stress may leave visible marks, even on your face, but be kind to the person you see in the mirror. Show her love, grace, and compassion. She needs it now more than ever.

Building resilience starts with a growth mindset, which means seeing challenges as opportunities to learn and grow rather than as obstacles. This approach helps you tackle problems with curiosity and creativity, leading to new solutions and skills. Gratitude is another key to resilience. Focusing on what you're thankful for can reframe tough experiences, helping you find positivity despite difficulties. Gratitude doesn't ignore problems but allows you to appreciate the good things in your life while addressing challenges. Positive reframing—choosing to see the silver linings in a situation—also strengthens emotional resilience over time. It helps reframe challenges as opportunities for growth, making it easier to navigate difficult moments.

Support networks are essential for building resilience. Reaching out to support groups or therapy can create a safe space to share your experiences and learn from others. Whether it's a local mom group or an online forum, connecting with other parents who understand your struggles can offer comfort and practical advice. Meeting other parents at the park, museums, or community events can create a sense of community and remind you that you're not alone.

Take the story of Tatiana, for example. After a difficult birth experience, she felt anxious and overwhelmed. At first, she struggled to process her emotions and felt isolated. But by joining a postpartum support group, she connected with mothers who had faced similar challenges. Their stories and encouragement helped her regain confidence and resilience. Eventually, Tatiana embraced her journey, finding joy in motherhood even amid obstacles. Her experience shows how powerful community and shared understanding can be.

Another example is Yesenia, who struggled with balancing work and motherhood after returning to her job from maternity leave. She felt torn between her responsibilities at work and home, battling guilt and exhaustion. Over time, Lisa developed strategies to manage her time more effectively and set boundaries to prioritize both her family and career. She learned to delegate tasks and integrate her roles rather than keeping them separate. Her resilience helped her succeed at work and home, proving that balance is possible with the right mindset and support.

Resilience isn't something you're born with—it's a skill you can build. By staying open to change, practicing gratitude, and leaning on your support system, you can develop the resilience you need to not only navigate motherhood but thrive in it. These strategies will help you handle challenges and empower you to grow in every area of your life.

In the next chapter, we will go over some of the things you can do to stop yourself from falling into the trap of self-doubt and comparison. We will also discuss how you can celebrate motherhood and find joy in the everyday moments, even when things feel overwhelming.

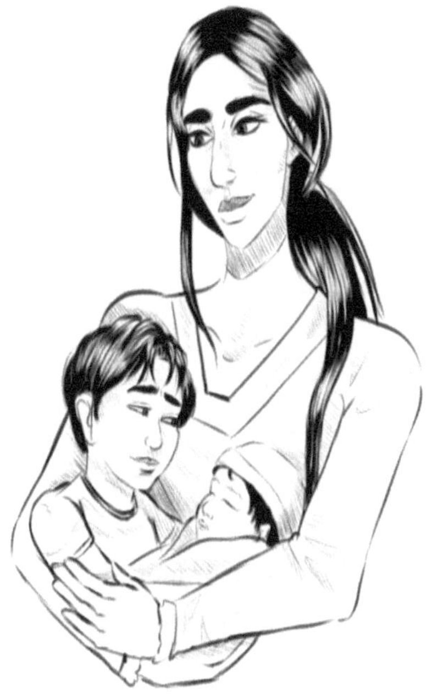

EXERCISE: BUILD YOUR PERSONALIZED SLEEP STRATEGY CHECKLIST

Objective: Create a checklist to streamline your nighttime routine and improve your rest.

Instructions:

1. **Step 1: Feeding Supplies**
   - List everything you need for nighttime feedings.

Example: bottles, formula pre-measured, water in bottles, mini fridge in the room.

____

____

____

2. **Step 2: Diaper Changing Essentials**
   - Write down items to keep near your bed for quick and easy diaper changes.

Example: diapers, wipes, diaper cream.

____

____

____

3. **Step 3: Sleep-Friendly Environment**
   - Identify the steps to create a calming sleep environment.

Example: use blackout curtains, white noise machine, dim nightlight.

____

____

____

4. **Step 4: Support Plan**
   - Outline how and when to seek support from family or professionals.

Example: schedule shifts with a partner, arrange help from a family member.

____

____

5. **Step 5: Personalize Your Checklist**
    - Combine the above steps into a personalized checklist that works for you.

Reflection:

After completing your checklist, reflect on how it can help simplify your routine and reduce nighttime stress. Keep it handy and adjust as needed!

CHAPTER 12
MOTHERHOOD

THE ULTIMATE ON-THE-JOB TRAINING

For each and every job I have had in my life, there is always a training period. A period where you learn the ins and outs of the job, gain experience, and develop skills to excel in that role. However, nothing could have prepared me for the ultimate on-the-job training – motherhood. Even with all the experience I had as a postpartum nurse, being a mother has been the most challenging and rewarding job I have ever had.

Let me paint a picture for you-you get thrown headfirst into the world of motherhood with little to no training. We as a society put so much emphasis on laboring and how to prepare for labor and just a tiny bit on all things postpartum. From the moment you hold your newborn in your arms, you are responsible for their every need – feeding, changing diapers, soothing cries, and everything in between. Some days, you'll feel like you've got everything under control, and other days, it might feel like you've failed. On the tough days—when you're tired, stressed, or not at your best—it's easy to feel defeated. Maybe you say or do something you regret and start doubting yourself.

But remember, one bad day doesn't define you.

In this chapter, we'll explore how you can prevent yourself from falling into the trap of self-doubt and how you can celebrate motherhood instead.

12.1 OVERCOMING SELF-DOUBT IN MOTHERHOOD

Parenthood is a journey filled with immense joy, but it also comes with moments where you don't feel like your best self. There may be times, even just 10 minutes a day, where you feel like you're failing or overreacting because you're overwhelmed and overstimulated.

But remember, you're learning too. Parenthood is a shared growth experience—you're raising each other. Every day, choose kindness toward yourself first. Give yourself grace. When you feel like you're about to lose your mind, take a moment to hug yourself and breathe.

A lot of unhealed emotions can surface unexpectedly during parenting. It's okay to not have all the answers. Stay flexible and give yourself permission to adapt as you go.

On tough days, whether it's you or your toddler struggling, try connecting. I often get close to my toddler and say, "I really want to start over. Can we start over? I'm sorry if I wasn't being very nice— I'm tired and overwhelmed. Let's take some deep breaths and maybe have a dance party to feel better. Will you join me?"

Then I tell him, "I love you so much. I'm so happy you're my baby, and I love being your mommy. I love you when I'm grumpy, and I love you when I'm sad."

Apologizing to your child is a beautiful thing. It shows them that you value them, that making mistakes is okay, and that we're all human. It's a powerful way to teach love, empathy, and imperfection.

The most important thing you can do in tough moments is take time to reflect and learn. Ask yourself what triggered your reaction, why it affected you, and how you can handle it differently next time. Parenthood is all about growth, and every challenge is an opportunity to improve. Be kind to yourself—just as you'd support a friend in the same situation. Focus on progress, not perfection. A tough day doesn't diminish the love and effort you give—it's just one piece in the parenthood puzzle.

As the early years fly by, you'll see how quickly your child grows and changes. One day, they're learning to hold their head up, and before long, they're taking their first steps. These milestones are amazing, but they also mean constant adaptation. Whether you're tackling baby sign language or cleaning up your toddler's yogurt art on the walls, each stage comes with its own highs and lows. Your ability to adjust is what makes it all work.

Understanding your child's developmental stages helps set realistic expectations. In the first months, they'll focus on motor and cognitive skills like grasping objects, following movement, and eventually sitting up. As they grow, emotional and social skills start to emerge—from their first smile to learning how to share, express feelings, and make friends. Recognizing these stages helps you create the right environment to support their growth. Each step is a chance for you both to learn and grow together.

There is an abundant amount of resources available to support you. Parenting books and guides offer practical tips, and online courses can deepen your understanding of child development. A resource I purchased and enjoyed is *"big little feelings"* and their course, "Winning the Toddler Stage." But you can also use websites like Mindset Works to provide advice on fostering a growth mindset—a belief that abilities can improve through practice and learning. This mindset is incredibly helpful as you navigate parenting, teaching your child essential skills like resilience and curiosity along the way.

A growth mindset isn't just for your child—it can also transform your parenting experience. View mistakes as opportunities to learn. For example, when your child gives the family cat an unexpected haircut, use it as a moment to teach empathy and responsibility. Celebrate small wins because every step forward is progress. This mindset encourages you to focus on the process, not just the outcome, and to find joy in learning and growing together.

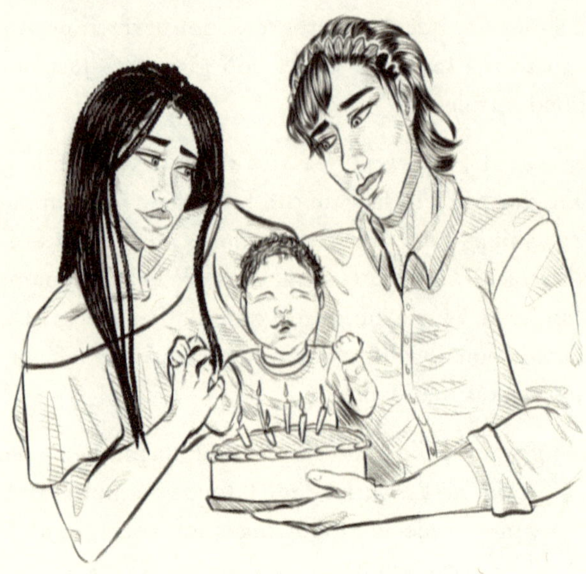

12.2 CELEBRATING THE MILESTONES

Imagine watching your child take their first steps—wobbly, determined, and full of curiosity. It's a moment that deserves more than just a quick photo for social media. Celebrating milestones, big or small, is about creating joy and motivation as a parent. These moments aren't just about marking time but appreciating growth. From your child's first words to milestones like potty training, every achievement deserves recognition. Each step is part of your child's unique developmental story.

One of the best parts of parenting is celebrating these moments with your child and family. Whether it's their first time eating on their own, saying "thank you," or learning a new skill, these milestones are worth the celebration. Sing a song, make music, or simply cheer them on—babies love positive reactions. They thrive on knowing their efforts are seen and appreciated. Show them that they're growing, that you notice their progress, and that they're becoming wiser and kinder every day.

Capturing these memories is also incredibly rewarding. I love taking photos and videos, but trust me; your phone fills up fast! To stay organized, try creating folders for specific themes like "First Words," "Milestones," or "Silly Moments." This makes it easier to revisit those special memories without feeling overwhelmed. Watching these moments on TV can also be magical—it brings those memories to life in a vivid way. If you're good at editing videos, try to do it soon after filming. If not, ask a tech-savvy friend or family member to help—it's a meaningful way for them to contribute, and you'll treasure the results.

You can also get creative with how you celebrate milestones. Consider making a scrapbook or journal filled with photos, notes, and little mementos from each moment. This becomes a keepsake that captures your journey together. Small family gatherings can also turn milestones into meaningful events. For example, if your child loves dinosaurs, throw a simple "Roar-some" party to celebrate their first word. It doesn't have to be elaborate—sometimes a picnic in the park is enough to make the moment special.

Celebrating these milestones has a real impact on your child's development. Positive reinforcement helps children build self-esteem and motivates them to keep trying, even when faced with challenges. By focusing on their effort and persistence rather than just the result, you teach them the value of hard work. This mindset encourages them to embrace new challenges with confidence, knowing their efforts are appreciated.

Many families create unique ways to celebrate achievements. One family I know hosts "milestone picnics" in their backyard. They toast each new achievement with lemonade and cupcakes, and everyone shares a memory or a wish for the child. Another family celebrates small daily wins at dinner, where each person shares something they're proud of that day—whether it's a toddler using a spoon or an older child finishing a puzzle. These small moments of recognition create a culture of celebration and gratitude within the family.

Celebrating milestones isn't just about recognizing progress—it's about building a sense of connection and belonging. Every moment, from the first babble to the first day of school, is a step in your child's journey. By celebrating these steps, you honor their growth and create lasting memories that strengthen family bonds. These moments become the stories you tell and the foundation of how your child understands love and achievement.

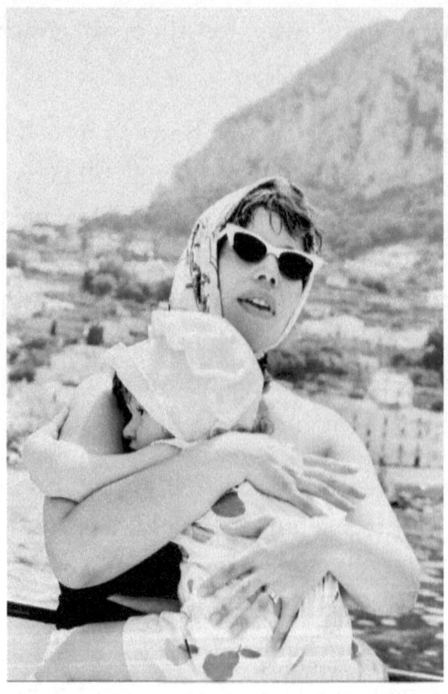

Me and Nikola — June 21, 2024 Capri, Italy | Photo by Eric Dilauro As a filmmaker, this is one of my favorite images ever captured. It's as if my vision board up leveled itself and created pure magic. Wearing my mother's vintage Hermès scarf—the same one I played dress-up with as a little girl—floating on a boat in Capri, fresh from a swim, holding my dream baby, giving thanks for this beautiful world.

12.3 THE TALES OF TRAVELING WITH CHILDREN

I know a lot of people hold the opinion that childbirth means the death of your passions. This is one thing I completely disagree with. Travel has always been a passion of mine, and becoming a parent hasn't changed that—it's only added a new layer of joy. At the time of writing this, my baby has been on 29 flights and just turned 29 months old (2 ½ years old). He absolutely loves the whole process of traveling, from arriving at the airport and checking in our bags to watching planes take off and land. He's even said "airplane" before his first birthday and delights in meeting pilots and peeking into cockpits.

Through our travels, he's learned so much. He understands different modes of transportation, picks up on the fact that people speak various languages, and has even mastered simple greetings in multiple tongues. He's always learning, and he does it with so much joy and curiosity. For us as parents, travel has become a way to bond, unwind, and introduce our child to the beauty and diversity of the world.

If you love to travel, my advice is simple: don't stop because you have children. Incorporate it into your life and make it part of your family's routine. Keep some structure while on the go—small, familiar rituals can go a long way in keeping things smooth. For example, no matter where we are, we always make time for a bath and bedtime stories before sleep. These little routines provide a sense of comfort and stability while still allowing for adventure. Traveling as a family has brought us closer and made us happier, more relaxed parents—and it can do the same for you.

And yes, there will be tough travel days. You may have a flight where your baby cries the entire time, and it feels like the longest journey of your life. But here's the thing: you can have hard days anywhere. On the 29 flights we've taken with my baby, only one was truly cringe-worthy. It was exhausting, and I tried my best not to stress about the return flight. To my surprise, the return flight was a dream—my baby played with toys and made friends with other kids on the plane. My motto during tough flights is simple: "This plane will land eventually, and it will all be worth it." Traveling with children isn't always easy, but the memories and experiences you create together make it all worthwhile.

12.4 FLEXIBILITY IN PARENTING

Parenting is all about adjusting to change. As children grow and develop, their needs shift quickly, and what worked yesterday might not work today. Being flexible means adapting your parenting style to meet these changes. It's about balancing structure, like routines and rules, with spontaneity, which encourages creativity and freedom. This balance creates a supportive environment where both you and your child can thrive.

One way to practice flexibility is through active listening—pay close attention to your child's words and actions to understand what they're feeling or needing. Kids don't always communicate verbally, so observing their behavior is key. Another strategy is allowing room for child-led activities. Let them choose a game to play or pick a bedtime book. This fosters independence and shows them their choices matter. It's not about losing control but empowering your child to have a voice.

Think of it this way - it can reduce stress and conflict. You'll argue less about rigid rules and find more creative solutions to challenges. For example, letting go of a strict schedule can make room for spontaneous outings or new adventures, bringing more joy and ease into your day-to-day life. This adaptability sharpens your problem-solving skills and helps you approach challenges with a calm, open mind.

Many parents have seen success by embracing flexibility. One mother switched to unschooling, a form of homeschooling that focuses on child-led learning, and her daughter thrived, developing a love for reading and science at her own pace. Another family adapted their routines to travel frequently, allowing their children to learn from new environments instead of sticking to rigid schedules.

Being flexible doesn't mean having no boundaries or structure. It's about creating a space where your family can grow and explore together. Letting go of the need for perfection can help you embrace the messy family life and appreciate its unpredictable moments. Flexibility encourages you to stay present, adapt, and enjoy the journey of raising your child, knowing that every day brings new experiences and opportunities.

12.5 CREATING YOUR LEGACY AS A MOTHER

Have you ever thought about the legacy you're creating with every hug, lullaby, and small decision? This legacy goes beyond traditions or values. It's built through your daily choices, shaping the story of your family. You define what matters most—whether it's family dinners, spontaneous adventures, or shared stories passed down through generations. Every decision helps build the environment your child grows up in, forming the foundation for their life. The values you emphasize serve as guiding principles for your family, offering direction even in difficult times.

Reflecting on the influence of your own maternal role models can be insightful. Perhaps your mother's quiet strength or your grandmother's resilience inspired your approach to parenting. These women, through their own unique experiences, have provided you with tools for your journey as a parent. Their influence is reflected in how you handle challenges, celebrate milestones, and nurture those around you. By reflecting on their impact, you can choose which lessons to carry forward and which traditions to redefine for your family. Acknowledging this influence allows you to be intentional about the legacy you want to create, one that reflects your family's evolving identity.

Being a mother is a powerful catalyst for personal growth. It challenges you in ways you might not have expected, reshaping your priorities and perspectives. As you adapt to this role, your aspirations often shift to accommodate your family's needs. This journey of self-discovery reveals strengths you didn't know you had.

Intentional parenting is about making thoughtful choices to create a meaningful legacy for your family. It involves setting long-term goals that align with your vision for your family and building a home rooted in love, growth, and learning. This might mean encouraging open communication, fostering curiosity, or teaching empathy and kindness. By aligning your daily actions with these goals, you create a nurturing environment where your children can thrive.

For some parents, this approach means consciously weaving their values and identity into their family life. One mother, for example, passed down her cultural heritage by incorporating traditional stories and recipes into her family's routines, connecting her children to their roots. Another family developed a mission statement to define their core values, using it as a guide for making decisions. This helped them stay grounded and focused during challenging times.

In the end, I leave you with a reminder to embrace your unique journey of motherhood and to create a legacy that reflects your family's values, beliefs, and identity. Be intentional in your parenting, and don't be afraid to redefine or break away from traditions that no longer serve you. By doing so, you are not only shaping the future of your family but also leaving behind a lasting impact for generations to come. You have the power to shape the world through the legacy you leave behind.

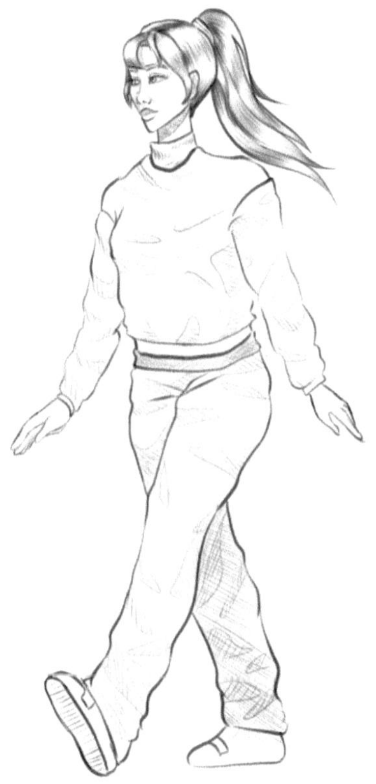

EXERCISE: GROWTH MINDSET REFLECTION

1. Think back to a recent parenting challenge you faced.

____

____

____

2. Reflect on how you handled the situation:

• What actions did you take?

____

____

• How did you feel during and after the challenge?

____

____

3. Write down your thoughts.

____

____

4. Identify lessons learned from the experience.

____

____

5. Consider how you can apply a growth mindset to similar
    challenges in the future.

____

____

Remember, parenting is a journey of constant learning. Each challenge is an opportunity to grow and strengthen your bond with your child. Take a moment to embrace this process, and remind yourself that perfection isn't the goal—growth is.

CONCLUSION

As we come to the end of "All Things Postpartum"," My intention is that these pages have offered you comfort and inspiration. Together, we've explored so many aspects of postpartum life, from physical recovery to the emotional ups and downs of new motherhood. We've covered breastfeeding basics, newborn care, relationships, and balancing work with family life. We've also emphasized the importance of self-care, discussed holistic approaches, and recognized diverse postpartum experiences. Above all, we've focused on building resilience throughout this journey.

The insights you've gained are a reminder of the strength within you. One key takeaway is the importance of building a supportive community. Creating your own "village" of friends, family, and fellow mothers can give you the understanding and help you need. Equally important is prioritizing self-care, practicing mindfulness, and embracing flexibility in parenting. These approaches can turn your postpartum experience into one of growth and empowerment. Lifelong learning in motherhood is essential—it gives you the tools to adapt and thrive as parenting evolves.

This book aims to shift the postpartum experience from being over-whelming to empowering and creative. It encourages you to view challenges as opportunities for growth and to have compassion for yourself when things don't go as planned. Embrace your journey with confidence and optimism. Let go of the pressure to be perfect and instead appreciate the beautiful chaos of motherhood. Remember, it's okay to ask for help, take a break, and celebrate small wins along the way.

Now is the time to take action. Use the tools and strategies discussed here. Find additional resources that resonate with you. Connect with communities that inspire and support you. Be open to learning and adapting as you navigate motherhood. Let curiosity and a desire for growth guide you, knowing that every step forward reflects your strength and resilience.

This book's vision is to celebrate the beauty and power of the postpartum journey. It's about education, inspiration, and empowerment. Carry this vision into your life and communities. Share your stories, support each other, and create spaces where every mother feels seen and valued. Together, we can change the narrative and celebrate motherhood in all its forms.

I want to express my deepest gratitude to you for being a part of this journey. Your courage to embrace motherhood fully is truly inspiring. Thank you for allowing this book to be a part of your postpartum experience. It's been an honor to walk alongside you, sharing stories and encouragement.

As we wrap up, remember this: you are capable, resilient, and strong. You have everything you need to face the ups and downs of motherhood. Trust yourself, lean on your tribe, and know you're never alone. Approach motherhood with an open heart and a sense of adventure. This is just the beginning of your story, full of opportunities for growth, love, and connection.

THANK YOU FOR BEING HERE

You made it.

You opened your heart, turned the pages, and chose yourself over and over again.

I hope you're walking away feeling more supported, more empowered, and more connected to the beautiful strength within you.

The world of postpartum needs more real conversations like this— and it grows stronger every time one of us shows up, shares, and lifts another mother higher.

HELP ANOTHER MOTHER FIND HER WAY

If this book encouraged you, supported you, or made you feel less alone, would you consider leaving a review?

- It takes less than a minute.
- It could make all the difference for a new mother searching for support.

Scan Here to go Directly to
the Review Page

Or visit:

https://www.amazon.com/review/create-review/?asin=B0F8526QZS

or simply leave a review wherever you purchased the book.

Your words could be the encouragement another mother needs to feel less alone and more supported.

Thank you for being part of this village. Together, we are rewriting what postpartum support looks like.

STAY CONNECTED + RECEIVE YOUR FREE GIFT

I would love to stay connected with you beyond these pages.

Download your free guide — The Gentle Postpartum Reset: www. johairamichelle.com/free

Follow along for daily inspiration and healing reflections:
TikTok: @allthingspostpartumbook
Website: www.johairamichelle.com

There's so much more ahead.

Let's keep growing — together.

With love and endless gratitude,
Johaira Michelle Dilauro, RN, BSN, CLE

REFERENCES

American College of Obstetricians and Gynecologists. (n.d.). Retrieved April 18, 2025, from https://acog.org

BMC Pregnancy and Childbirth. (n.d.). Retrieved April 18, 2025, from https://bmcpregnancychildbirth.biomedcentral.com

Calm. (n.d.). Retrieved April 18, 2025, from https://calm.com

Calzada, E. J., Fernandez, Y., & Cortes, D. E. (2010). Incorporating the cultural value of respeto into a framework of Latino parenting. *Cultural Diversity and Ethnic Minority Psychology, 16*(1), 77–86. https://doi.org/10.1037/a0016071

Centers for Disease Control and Prevention. (n.d.). Retrieved April 18, 2025, from https://cdc.gov

Cleveland Clinic. (2022, February 28). What is gentle parenting? *Cleveland Clinic*. https://health.clevelandclinic.org/what-is-gentle-parenting

Cultural Atlas. (n.d.). Indian culture – Family. *SBS*. Retrieved April 18, 2025, from https://culturalatlas.sbs.com.au/indian-culture/indian-culture-family

DONA International. (n.d.). Retrieved April 18, 2025, from https://dona.org

Dr. Noze Best. (n.d.). Retrieved April 18, 2025, from https://drnozebest.com

Ergobaby. (n.d.). Retrieved April 18, 2025, from https://ergobaby.com

Forbes. (n.d.). Retrieved April 18, 2025, from https://forbes.com

Frontiers in Psychology. (n.d.). Retrieved April 18, 2025, from https://frontiersin.org

Healthline. (n.d.). Retrieved April 18, 2025, from https://healthline.com

High Country Doulas. (n.d.). Retrieved April 18, 2025, from https://highcountrydoulas.com

Hinds, S. (2021, March 30). It takes a village to raise a child—African proverb: Here's why it's true. *Medium*. https://medium.com/@sherlaine.hinds/it-takes-a-village-to-raise-a-child-african-proverb-heres-why-it-s-true-53122b998801

HuffPost. (n.d.). Retrieved April 18, 2025, from https://huffpost.com

Lancaster General Health. (n.d.). Retrieved April 18, 2025, from https://lancastergeneralhealth.org

Mahmee. (n.d.). Retrieved April 18, 2025, from https://mahmee.com

Makemake Organics. (n.d.). Retrieved April 18, 2025, from https://makemakeorganics.com

Mayo Clinic Health System. (n.d.). Retrieved April 18, 2025, from https://mayoclinichealthsystem.org

Medium. (n.d.). Retrieved April 18, 2025, from https://medium.com

Mind Made Well. (n.d.). Retrieved April 18, 2025, from https://mindmadewell.com

Mindset Works. (n.d.). Retrieved April 18, 2025, from https://mindsetworks.com

My First Nursery. (n.d.). Why do Scandinavian parents nap their babies outside in cold temperatures? *My First Nursery*. Retrieved April 18, 2025, from https://myfirstnursery.co.uk/blogs/news/why-do-scandinavian-parents-nap-their-babies-outside-in-cold-temperatures

NHS Start for Life. (n.d.). Retrieved April 18, 2025, from https://nhs.uk

NPR. (n.d.). Retrieved April 18, 2025, from https://npr.org

National Association for the Education of Young Children. (n.d.). Retrieved April 18, 2025, from https://naeyc.org

National Institutes of Health – PMC. (n.d.). Retrieved April 18, 2025, from https://pmc.ncbi.nlm.nih.gov

Office on Women's Health. (n.d.). Retrieved April 18, 2025, from https://womenshealth.gov

Parents Editors. (2022, May 19). What is helicopter parenting? *Parents*. https://www.parents.com/parenting/better-parenting/what-is-helicopter-parenting/

Psychology Today. (n.d.). Retrieved April 18, 2025, from https://psychologytoday.com

PubMed. (n.d.). Retrieved April 18, 2025, from https://pubmed.ncbi.nlm.nih.gov

ScienceDirect. (n.d.). Retrieved April 18, 2025, from https://sciencedirect.com

Sears, W., & Sears, M. (n.d.). What is attachment parenting? *AskDrSears.com*. Retrieved April 18, 2025, from https://www.askdrsears.com/topics/parenting/attachment-parenting/

Sleep Foundation. (n.d.). Retrieved April 18, 2025, from https://sleepfoundation.org

Spirit Codex. (n.d.). Husband Having a Girlfriend: Spiritual Meaning and Insights for Personal Growth. Retrieved April 18, 2025, from https://spiritcodex.net/husband-having-a-girlfriend-spiritual-meaning/

The Bump. (n.d.). Retrieved April 18, 2025, from https://thebump.com

The Family Center. (n.d.). Retrieved April 18, 2025, from https://thefamilycenterfc.org

U.S. Breastfeeding Committee. (n.d.). Retrieved April 18, 2025, from https://usbreastfeeding.org

Verywell Health. (n.d.). Retrieved April 18, 2025, from https://verywellhealth.com

What to Expect. (n.d.). Retrieved April 18, 2025, from https://whattoexpect.com

Wikipedia contributors. (n.d.). Amae. *Wikipedia*. Retrieved April 18, 2025, from https://en.wikipedia.org/wiki/Amae

Wildflower Health. (n.d.). Retrieved April 18, 2025, from https://wildflowerllc.com

Writing Mindset. (n.d.). Retrieved April 18, 2025, from https://writingmindset.org

Yasharoff, H. (2025, April 15). Kristen Bell and Dax Shepard embrace free-range parenting. *USA Today*. https://www.usatoday.com/story/life/health-wellness/2025/04/15/dax-shepard-kristen-bell-free-ra

ABOUT THE AUTHOR

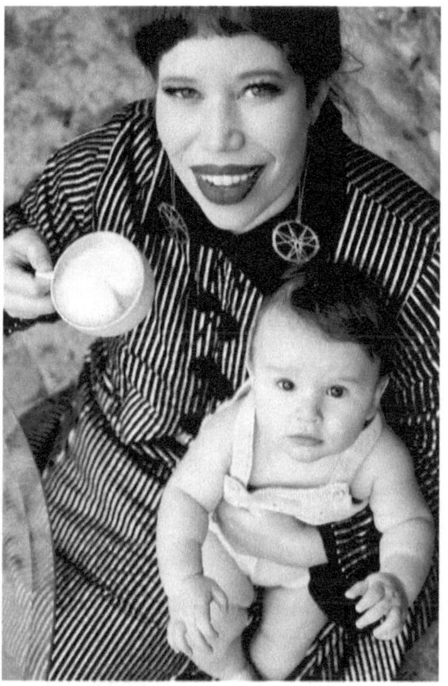

Me and Nikola — February 8, 2023 Los Angeles, CA | Photo by Jonathan Christian Fernandez My community came together to help me capture this sacred six-month chapter of motherhood. What you don't see: the early morning makeup run, the hope that Nikola would nap in the car, and the full-blown car seat meltdown. Nothing went as planned—except this smile. And that smile says it all: I was so happy.

Johaira Michelle Dilauro, RN, BSN, CLE is a registered nurse with over a decade of experience supporting families through the transformative postpartum journey. Her clinical background in maternal health is the foundation for a broader mission: to heal, inspire, and elevate through creativity and community.

A multidisciplinary artist and the founder of Artist Wellness Day, Johaira curates' immersive experiences that combine live music, motivational speakers, meditation, nourishing food, and joyful dance —all in service of healing and connection.

As a filmmaker, she creates bold, advocacy-driven stories that often blend her scientific expertise with deeply expressive art. Her original music—quirky, bilingual, and rooted in themes of community and resilience—speaks to both personal and collective experiences, including the pandemic era.

She also designs unique costumes for her music videos in collaboration with seamstress, and her photography captures both avant-garde style and everyday soul.

Johaira is also a state board-certified esthetician, bringing a deep understanding of skin health and holistic care into her broader wellness approach.

Her work as a public speaker and event curator centers on community wellness, and her passion for global travel informs much of her visual and narrative art.

She feels most alive when dancing on the beach, traveling the world, capturing beauty through her lens, or dreaming up her next big idea.

She is a proud director, producer, and actress—equally at home behind the camera as she is in front of it.

Above all, Johaira is an emerging entrepreneur with a vision: to build a magical, intentional, and fully creative life—one bold project at a time.

You can connect with Johaira, explore more healing resources, and join the growing community at:

TikTok: @allthingspostpartumbook
Website: www.johairamichelle.com